"I am so glad Dr. J manifested his *Manifesto*. There is so much in here, yet it's a thin enough [illegible] not be intimidating. Take what he says to heart and watch yourself become [illegible] humane human."

Erich Schiffmann
Author of "YOGA: The Spirit and Practice of Moving into Stillness"

"Oftentimes, we see the world from within our own box — it's human nature. We have to work at it to examine the edges, the corners, the boundaries and see which parts of whatever point of view we're holding actually serve us and promote health and well-being. Dr. Jeremy Brook has done just that — examined fully the box of chiropractic (including the founding principles of the scientific art) and the box of Yoga, and the bigger box of the human body, as well as what it means to be really healthy. His keen sensibility, sharp mind and inquisitive spirit have penned a manifesto that offers something profound and meaningful for the reader to contemplate, and use as a springboard to question the status quo of mainstream medical information that we're given and instead, to actually explore what good health really means and how we can cultivate it. The enthusiasm with which Dr. Brook writes is palpable and his carefully thought-out ideas and syntheses of traditions will spark self-inquiry. He'll inspire belief in chiropractic if you're a skeptic and encourage you to try a Yoga practice appropriate to your body and situation. The Spinechecker's Manifesto is a testament to Dr. Jeremy Brook, to the complementary sciences of chiropractic and Yoga and is a welcome addition to current thoughts on health. And…you can't help but smile as you read it; Dr. Brook's lively voice offers up ideas that make this worthy of returning to its pages again and again."

Felicia Marie Tomasko, RN
Editor-in-Chief, LA YOGA Ayurveda and Health Magazine
President, California Association of Ayurvedic Medicine
Member, Board of Directors, National Ayurvedic Medical Association

"I thoroughly enjoyed the easy read of Dr. Brook's book. An inspirational manifesto that provides insightful information about chiropractic. Dr. Brook brings to light how complementary and essential yoga is to chiropractic for maintaining a healthy and flexible spine."

June Leslie Wieder, D.C.
Chiropractor and author of "Song of The Spine"

"Dr. Jeremy Brook's *The Spinechecker's Manifesto* is a wonderful contribution to chiropractic literature and human potential. It links the truths from the wisdom traditions to common sense wisdom and chiropractic principles! Well done!"

Simon A. Senzon, MA, DC
Author of "Chiropractic Foundations, The Secret History of Chiropractic, and The Spiritual Writings of B.J. Palmer"

THE SPINECHECKER'S MANIFESTO

DRUG-FREE SECRETS TO PAIN-FREE LIVING, MORE ENERGY, ANTI-AGING, & BETTER SLEEP

CREDITS & COPYRIGHTS

ISBN 978-1-329-30797-1

THE SPINECHECKER'S MANIFESTO:
Drug-Free Secrets to Pain-Free Living, More Energy, Anti-Aging, & Better Sleep

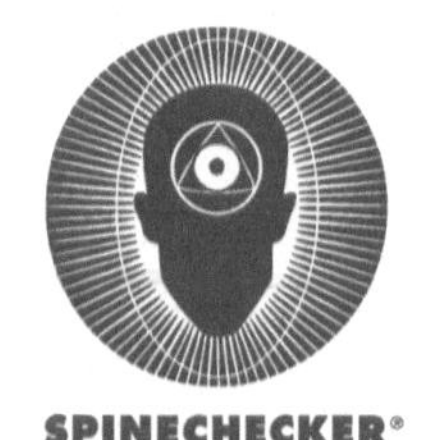

Original Spinechecker logo was created by Sean Odell in 2004.

Art Credits

Cover and pages 72-73 Copyright© 2009 by Robert Sturman

Illustrations Copyright© by Dr. Joe Ventura of www.posturepro.com & anatomyworld.com on the following pages:
10, 17, 18-19, 21, 25-26, 28, 32, 45-46, 48-49

Spinechecker Superhero on page 56 by Shannan Burkley.
Shannan is a visual artist for movies such as X-Men: The Last Stand, Fantastic Four: Rise of the Silver Surfer, Australia,The Golden Compass, Master and Commander: The Far Side of the World, and more.

Medical Disclaimer

The information provided in this manifesto is of a general nature and cannot substitute for the advice of a health professional (for instance, a qualified doctor of chiropractic or medical doctor/ physician).

You are encouraged to consult your doctor of chiropractic, or your medical doctor to obtain professional advice, who may agree or disagree with the information and materials contained in this book.

This book makes no promises of reaching enlightenment.

D = *this symbol appears beside words that will have a definition provided in the glossary*

DEDICATION

For my grandparents: Abraham, Gabe, Irene, and Naomi

INDEX

ABOUT DR. JEREMY BROOK, THE "SPINECHECKER"™

The Turning Point

Life is full of little tiny crises. You know. Your boss had a temper blow up. The baby had a bad restless night of sleep. The car needs a sudden repair. Working at a desk has brought back pain and wrist pain. The new loan for your business didn't go through, or your bank account is overdrawn. Whatever it is you are going through, there is a way to get on top of it, find your center, and feel great. I know, it can be overwhelming sometimes and you can feel as though there is no way to find any sort of center, or even think about feeling great. But the truth is, if you keep going the way you are going, you might never get around to feeling great. You need guidance, even wisdom, from someone who knows how to get you from your worst to your best so that you are prepared to handle anything that life throws at you.

Greetings! My name is Dr. Jeremy Brook, "The Spinechecker." I own The Life Center Chiropractic in Los Angeles, a unique center that incorporates the disciplines of traditional chiropractic with yoga, where I adjust patients every day who are suffering from chronic back pain, fatigue, arthritis, insomnia, low sex drive, poor digestion, and so much more. And every week I see these people get better under my care, and even completely heal themselves from the inside out. My philosophy is integrated into my work, and because it is so successful, I was encouraged by those around me to write a book to help patients and other chiropractors utilize what I have discovered to be true about energy, healing, and health in their own lives. Because it works.

My healing philosophy lets you connect with your inborn intelligence, the same force that is beating your heart and growing your hair right now, to optimize your healing potential and creative talents and basically just feel great every day. My perspective stems from a background of yoga, music, college athletics, and biology, but it is also coupled with my own personal experiences that include: numerous sports injuries, a car accident on the 405 Freeway, and good old-fashion emotional stress. My desire is to help you create a body that is strong, flexible, and adaptable to the stresses of living in a fast-paced, technologically advanced civilization.

See, when I was eight years old, I received my first chiropractic adjustment. Not for back pain or one of any other different ailments, but because my dad knew the importance of maintaining a healthy spine through my developing years. My dad loved chiropractic and actually considered going to chiropractic school. But that wasn't to be his path... it was to be mine. In essence, he groomed me to be his personal chiropractor. Since the third grade, all I desired to be when I grew up was a chiropractor. Flash forward twelve years later, while playing rugby at the University of California at Irvine, in the second to last game of the season I sustained a separated shoulder and broken nose. Early in the game while making a tackle, I took a knee to my left shoulder that changed the course of my life. To add insult to injury, I stayed in the game, only to break my nose in the second half. Well that simple tackle ended up separating my shoulder and misaligned a couple bones in my neck. Talk about pain! I couldn't lift my arm more than a few inches from my side and now my nose was repositioned on the opposite side of my face. Since we had a physical therapist who sponsored our rugby team, I went to him to check out my separated shoulder. Well, after a year and a half of physical therapy treatments, I became extremely depressed that my pain hadn't resolved and I could still hardly move my shoulder.

Since the physical therapy treatments consisting of muscle stimulation, ultrasound, exercises, and massage, hadn't resolved my problem, my next step was a visit to the orthopedist, who said surgery would be a good option. I was given Vicodin to deal with the pain until we could set a date for surgery. God bless the Vicodin, because while on spring break, I had a horrifically painful reaction to it that it landed me in the emergency room with crippling abdominal pain. The only position comfortable for me was to curl up in a tight ball and not move. At the hospital I received a pink milk-like cocktail and in about an hour or so I was back on my feet. Thank God for those emergency room doctors!

After being released from the hospital, something inside me told me to go to the chiropractor. I went back to my first-ever chiropractor, Dr. Paul Weber, who I hadn't seen in years, to get checked out. He took X-rays, motion palpated my spine and found the cause of my problem. Dr. Weber delivered a specific adjustment to my atlas, the top

ABOUT DR. JEREMY BROOK, THE "SPINECHECKER"™ *(cont.)*

vertebrae and the first thoracic vertebrae, and I was given my life back. My shoulder wasn't even adjusted, just my spine! I wasted a year and a half of my life struggling with pain. In one miracle adjustment I was eighty percent better! Over the course of a few months I continued to receive adjustments and my shoulder pain was a thing of the past. I did have surgery though... on my nose... to reposition it back on the center of my face.

My Discovery

Having put the gladiator sports behind me, like rugby and boxing, (oh yeah.... I also had a dream of being the Jewish version of Ray "Boom Boom" Mancini, who happens to be a friend and chiropractic patient) any activity that did not involve risk of injury seemed attractive. While leaving the gym one night I saw some people walking with yoga mats toward the exercise room. I followed them and set up at the back of class. I had no idea what to expect when I went to my first yoga class in 1996. I innately knew I needed to stretch out my banged up body and I figured yoga was good place to start. There I was sitting in my first yoga class, with no mat, and still wearing my sneakers. (Side note: For those of you who don't do yoga, yoga is traditionally practiced barefoot.)

My journey into yoga began in the Sivananda yoga tradition, which was unique considering the gym setting. Most classes at gyms these days have more of a "power" or athletic attitude. This one was super chill and non-competitive. A typical class consisted of a full range of yoga postures with bansuri flute music playing in the background. To be honest, I was the tightest person in the class! But there was something magical that I felt when stretching, breathing, and concentrating on the energy centers in my body. My love for yoga was born. My friends couldn't believe their eyes, especially when I would miss watching Los Angeles Lakers games to practice yoga. Because at the time yoga hadn't become mainstream, so even my family thought I had suffered too many head traumas from rugby.

I graduated from UC Irvine in 1996 with a degree in biology, and entered Palmer College of Chiropractic-West, one of the world's most prestigious chiropractic schools. It was there that I earned the Virgil V. Strang Award for philosophical excellence in my graduating class. It was at Palmer-West that I discovered how deep chiropractic science really is. I had no idea before I studied it, that chiropractic is not just a science and an art, but is also a vitalistic discipline. Sure chiropractic got me out

ABOUT DR. JEREMY BROOK, THE "SPINECHECKER"™ *(cont.)*

of pain, but chiropractic transcends pain relief. It has a mind-blowing philosophy that is unique among the health care professions in that it recognizes the relationship between structure, function, performance and the expression of health.

During this period of time, I awakened to new age and old school philosophy and explored other styles of yoga such as Bikram and vinyasa yoga. The combination of yoga and chiropractic was cracking my body wide open both physically and mentally. As a result of the wisdom teachings, I began to incorporate yoga along with chiropractic adjustments in a supportive manner. The primordial yoga sequences I designed and showed my patients helped them hold their adjustments. I felt I was definitely onto something. Thankfully my chiropractic school mentor, Dr. Mindy Pelz-Hall, allowed me to explore this combination while practicing in her office. The sequences I put together for the cervical spine, the Cervical Salutations, were designed under her roof! Thanks again, Dr. Mindy!

In 2001, I returned to Los Angeles to open The Life Center Chiropractic, a unique healing oasis that incorporates specific scientific chiropractic adjustments with yoga. It was a dream come true. I had the opportunity to take care of Olympic athletes, NBA players, boxing champions, movie stars, prolific writers and directors, pregnant women, martial artists and yoga masters!

My yoga practice elevated during the next several years as I became a dedicated student of Ashtanga yoga. Unfortunately the combination of postures in Ashtanga's regimented sequence didn't work well for me at the time. Perhaps it was because my body was still so tight and I was practicing yoga for two hours at 6 am in the morning. Tight baseline body + stiff in the morning = hard practice. So I shifted gears and designed my own style and practice that took into consideration my occupation as a chiropractor, my past injuries and limitations, and my emotional constitution. With the influence of Bruce Lee combined with Dr. Arno Burnier's chiropractic training program, I refined a body-mind training system for myself that includes rubber band speed training, indo board balance training, weight training, and a chiropractic-specific yoga sequence, that will be available on DVD.

In 2008, I became a Certified Chiropractic Wellness Practitioner (C.C.W.P.) through the International Chiropractic Association Council on Wellness Science. This practical

ABOUT DR. JEREMY BROOK, THE "SPINECHECKER"™ *(cont.)*

research- and science-based program, designed by wellness genius Dr. James Chestnut, addresses important health issues such as wellness-based nutrition/ hygiene, wellness-based exercise/fitness, and wellness-based stress reduction/positive mental attitude development. This program gave me more scientific validation about the link between the spine, the nervous system, and total health than I could have dreamed of (Buy his books immediately if you are looking for an endless amount of scientific references that support the ancient books of yoga). As a result of this program, my understanding of the human body has never been stronger.

Recently, while practicing yoga I received a strong epiphany to learn to play the sitar. Ancient civilizations believed that music had great power of healing. I was reminded of Apollo, the patron god of medicine and healing, music, poetry, and archery, as well as traditional Chinese martial arts. Traditional Chinese martial arts training placed as much emphasis on nurturing the spirit as it did on the fighting ability of the aspiring student. Many of the greatest figures in martial arts history were as renowned as healers as they were as warriors. I've learned firsthand that the human body is like a musical instrument, expressing numerous frequencies and rhythms. Tuning the spine, or playing the sitar, brings us back to order and sets into motion a pattern that attunes us to our natural healthy beat.

Amazingly, my epiphany came to life as I am currently taking lessons from sitar virtuoso Ustad Nishat Khan! In fact, you'll find that music is a central theme throughout this manifesto.

The most important lesson I've learned in my short time on this planet is that your commitment to health starts by reading scientific journals, books, and manifestos... and then you have to go out there and do the work.

So get moving and playing! It will be more fun and less painful!

FOREWARD

This manifesto was written for several people in mind. It was written for my brothers and sisters in the chiropractic profession, the chiropractic patient, the yoga teacher, other health care practitioners, and lifestyle enthusiasts.

This is a manifesto that contains a general recipe for living a healthy life. Suggested movement, stretching, strengthening, breathing, and concentrating sequences are provided, along with basic guides for healthy eating, sleeping, and stress reduction. One major point to consider is that we individually have a unique body-mind constitution, much like a fingerprint. This manifesto respects the fact that we have different physical bodies in size, shape, strength, and flexibility, as well as different emotional appetites.

But as members of the animal kingdom we have specific lifestyle requirements if we want to be healthy, or maybe, strive to be an enlightened being. The human species is complicated, yet simple. We need to get the physical body in alignment with the mental body, the mental body in alignment with the intellectual body, and the intellectual body in alignment with the spiritual body. Thankfully, great wisdom teachers of past and present have given us information on how to achieve such balance through a holistic body-mind-spirit approach.

"Intention is paramount."

Arno Burnier, D.C.

Despite our many differences, each of us has an optimum state on a physical, emotional, mental, social, sexual, and psychic level, as well as a range of limitations. The goal of this manifesto is to help you maximize your 'self' by knowing your strengths and limitations. With that self-knowledge, we have a baseline to build upon.

Self-knowledge begins with awareness. According to the yogic sages, there are 4 obstacles to attaining super-awesome health and happiness. Here they are:

1. Suffering

2. Pessimism

3. Instability of the Body

4. Irregularity of the Breath

By conquering these obstacles we set the stage for experiencing bliss. This manifesto has an underlying goal of increasing bliss and vitality by removing interference from our nervous system. Through impeccable motion and alignment the breath is able to flow freely, the body becomes strong; and negative thoughts, stress, and tension dissolve, which then leads to diminished suffering. The end result, or effect of the removal of interference, is the bliss state.

If created properly, this manifesto will serve as a transformational experience that will align our body, mind and spirit. We will learn how to scan and listen to our body and develop a deeper relationship to our 'self' on all levels. It is an empowering and life-affirming experience that will help propel us to the next level in our life journey.

Sometimes we're going to get knocked out like a UFC fighter and we may need a new strategy to get back on our feet! This manifesto is for the person who just got knocked out as well as for the champion who wants to stay on top. This may mean getting rid of stiff joints, asthma, aching backs, constipation, or infertility, or keeping your immunity at its highest level.

GIVE YOUR LIFE SOME "STYLE"

INCORPORATING THE DISCIPLINES OF CHIROPRACTIC & YOGA

"Move it!

Stretch it!

Strengthen it!

Energize it!"

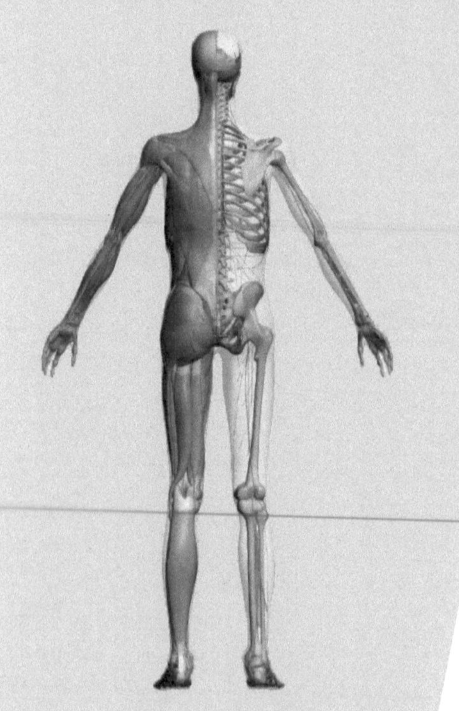

Dr. Jeremy Brook

I'm often asked how I am able to incorporate the disciplines of chiropractic and yoga. I view chiropractic and yoga as virtual brothers and sisters. They are siblings who push evolution and consciousness to new heights (and the chiropractors and yogis are leading the way on this path!).

The correlation between chiropractic and yoga is the spine. Both disciplines recognize that correct alignment, structural integrity, and the health of the nervous system are conducive to better health on physical, psychological and spiritual levels. As we already know, by freeing the energies of the spine, the tissues of the entire body are better controlled by the higher centers of the brain since messages can travel unimpeded. The organs of the body benefit, and their internal function is synergistically enhanced.

Chiropractic took the gross manipulation of the body - a practice also found in yoga - and created a science around a "specific adjustment" of the spinal bones. Chiropractic as we define it today was discovered in 1895, and has evolved to new heights as advanced technology has became available. The use of X-rays, infrared thermography, surface electromyography, electroencephalogram (EEG), and other stress response tests, as well as computerized range of motion studies have equipped today's chiropractor with a sophisticated set of instruments, along with hands-on palpation, to accurately diagnose and correct distortions or misalignments of the spine, called vertebral subluxation, that cause nerve interference.

Originally I began studying yoga in an effort to recover from rugby injuries. Two years later I started chiropractic school and merged the two like peanut butter and chocolate! The combination was powerful and helped me develop as a healer and human. In my experience, yoga and chiropractic adjustments have had profound benefits on my own health as well as on the health of my patients. I have been practicing yoga for over 15 years, and have been a student of many yoga styles. I recognize the yoga/chiropractic combination appears to be unmatched when it comes to results on a body-mind level.

My personal philosophy goes something like this: Unlock the spine first to take the pressure off the nervous system. This is done with a specific scientific chiropractic adjustment based on the individual situation. Then, it's essential to move with intelligence to make sure the released energy (also known as chi, in Chinese medicine, or prana in Sanskrit, the language of the yoga tradition) gets deposited in the right place and in the right concentration. That's where yoga works wonders! A person is able to move without restriction to access their sacred geometry, hopefully without pain and suffering. I see the chiropractic adjustment as a precursor to yoga. Chiropractic helps unlock a spinal bone or bones that are stuck and jammed. Once it is "freed up", appropriate yoga practice ensures that the joint moves freely through all ranges of motion. To maintain that range of motion, awareness, and intelligence on a day-to-day basis, yoga and chiropractic reigns supreme!

For a lasting effect, a chiropractic adjustment often needs to be accompanied by postural corrections, such as cervical traction, mind-body education, and changes in habitual patterns. We are always sequencing from one movement to another, from the moment we get out of bed, as we flow through the activities of our day. Life happens better with as few glitches as possible. When a patient seeks care at The Life Center Chiropractic, we do a thorough evaluation to determine what the architecture looks like. Once a protocol of care has been established, we begin with an adjusting and movement sequence program. Later, when damaged joints have been restored to their natural state, cervical traction and other back-bending props are introduced to stretch the contracted ligaments and restore curves where they have been either reversed or straightened. Integrating specific vinyasa[D]/movement/stretching/strengthening patterns are also encouraged to re-educate the body to attain a stronger and more flexible spine.

The union of chiropractic and yoga allows for a supremely integrated modern human!

At The Life Center Chiropractic, we offer workshops such as Spinal Wellness, "Holistic Approach to Dealing with Stress", and Wellness Nutrition. I also serve as a guest instructor for teacher training programs around California teaching Yogic Anatomy, The Neurology of Yoga, and Yoga as a Key Player in the Wellness Revolution. Basically, I enlighten yogis and teachers on the biomechanical and energetic nature of human anatomy and physiology, especially the spine. I find that many yoga instructors are knowledgeable in asana[D]/postures, but lack a corresponding understanding of anatomy. We all have different bodymind constitutions that don't necessarily fit into one category. Some "final shape" asanas or postures may never happen because one's architecture isn't designed to move in that manner. Thus, I created a curriculum for yogis and yoga teachers to teach how the

"Keep it simple:

1. Get your spine checked

2. Eat healthy

3. Sleep well

4. Exercise smart

5. Think good thoughts

6. Love with all your might"

Dr. Jeremy Brook

GIVE YOUR LIFE SOME "STYLE"

INCORPORATING THE DISCIPLINES OF CHIROPRACTIC & YOGA *(cont.)*

body moves from a chiropractic standpoint. It was while teaching Yogic Anatomy that the concept of the manifesto was born. The intention is to provide you with suggested "do's and don'ts" following an adjustment to make sure the released energy was properly and effectively integrated. The goal is to move with intelligence and ease to enhance coordination among the brain and the spinal cord, spinal nerves, tissues and cells; and then, from the tissue and cell back to the brain. Specific geometric movements and breathing techniques, borrowed from the yogic traditions in a nondogmatic manner, are illustrated and emphasized in this manual. Since every person has their own unique blueprint, this manifesto will provide you with archetypal poses to facilitate healthy movement and physiology.

It is my hope this manifesto speaks to you and brings forth great health and abundance in your life.

"Actively create a ritual toward personal growth."

MY VISION

It is my passion to serve active lifestyle enthusiasts looking to possess a powerful, energy-efficient and strain-free body-mind though chiropractic and yoga.

It is my vision to adjust as many people as divinely possible, and to educate them about strategies to tap into their innate healing ability.

It is also my vision to transform our current health consciousness and paradigm from one that is dependent on prescription drugs, inappropriate surgeries, and any method that seeks to treat or mask the symptom to one focused on caring for the entire individual by correcting and preventing the underlying cause.

I achieve this by creating a space that honors the inborn wisdom of men and women, and I call it The Life Center Chiropractic, offering the most respectful and honoring chiropractic technique in the profession, with yoga and lifestyle strategies to optimize one's total health.

I also achieve my vision through my teaching of ancient concepts of life force and holistic healing, to optimize vitality, and teach methods that release stress and promote balance.

It is my goal to ensure that the impulse generated in the brain for the body travels without restriction so that this impulse can be heard clearly, felt deeply and ultimately acted upon.

"I have answered the time-worn question — what is life?": "The dualistic system — spirit and body — united by intellectual life — the soul — is the basis of this science of biology."

Dr. D.D. Palmer

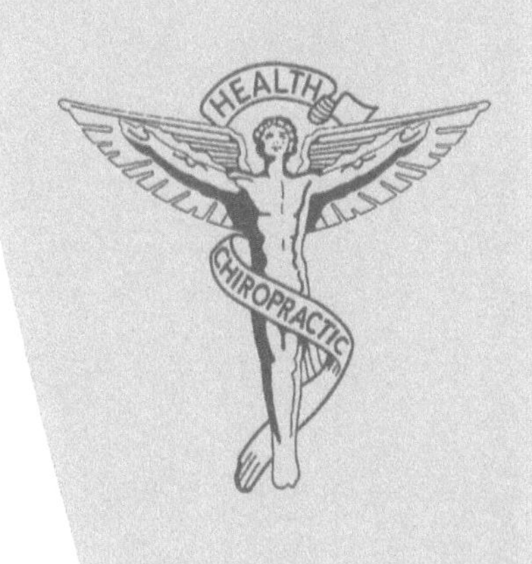

THE GOLDEN AGE OF HEALTH

I imagine a world where chiropractic constitutes a foundational system in mankind's quest for total health.

I imagine a world where people revolt like the French Revolution against the dogmatic and dangerous overuse of prescription drugs and unnecessary surgery, and move toward natural healing methods. Shortcuts to health through the use of painkillers, muscle relaxers, tranquilizers, and other concoctions are replaced by a deep thirst for getting to the root cause of dis-ease...correcting it...and then maintaining it!

"The doctor of the future will give no medicine but will interest his patients in the care of the human frame, in diet and in the cause and prevention of disease."

Thomas Edison

I imagine a world where a holistic body-mind-training program is practiced by every man, woman, and child based on their own unique body-mind-constitution.

Chiropractors, acupuncturists, old-school osteopaths, ayurvedic doctors, and yoga teachers are the new health maintaining organization. I imagine a world where health care providers view the spine as the centerpiece of the health foundation. Caring for the structural infrastructure and the flow of innate nerve energy.

Medical doctors are the experts in emergency care.

I imagine a world where television drug commercials are a thing of the past, just like cigarette commercials.

I imagine a world where the foods we eat are from the earth are not altered and aren't packaged with labels with unpronounceable words.

I imagine a world where people listen to their innate intelligence and strengthen their minds and bodies just like the ancients.

I imagine a world where this wellness revolution was swift and complete. Maybe this is what the Mayas meant by the end of the world, as we know it: The end of the separation between mind and body and the delivery of a vital united human species.

THE CHIROPRACTIC LIFESTYLE

To remain in a state of balance and optimal health is a skill not known by most people in our fast-paced, technologically-advanced society. The secret to health lies in developing a holistic body-mind training program that addresses all of our innate requirements.

The physical components of looking after one's biosphere are plentiful. Our choices include yoga, weight training, cardiovascular training, and more. But the physical component is incomplete if not balanced by pure, live, organic foods, a positive mental outlook, a spiritual practice, and rest and recuperation. Only when our traumas, toxins, and negative thoughts are reduced can we keep ourselves in a state of balance with our surrounding environment.

D.D. Palmer, who founded the science, art, and philosophy of chiropractic, wrote about an inborn intelligence that lies within us all. This innate intelligence is imbedded into our DNA, orchestrates our healing processes, and allows us to strive toward optimal health. Cellular youth, however, is only with us until the age of 30, when our bio-machine begins to show wear and tear. After all, we are under gravity's constant pressure, not to mention the stresses of a Western industrialized lifestyle. Our innate healing abilities become challenged and sometimes strained if we don't access the required resources to keep this intelligence flowing.

"Chiropractic is a natural health care discipline based on philosophical and scientific principles that emphasize the body's innate ability to heal itself without drugs or surgery."

We have an active choice in our decisions that determine whether we will express balance and health, or slide toward decay and degeneration. The key is to cultivate a plan to minimize damage and preserve our bodies as long as possible. With a holistic body-mind training program we are able to combat the unnatural as well as the natural stresses of life, allowing our innate intelligence to flow without interference, while undoing much of the unwelcome effects of accelerated aging.

If we stay in the center, we never have to find it. Health is easier to maintain if we know and practice the laws of keeping the body mind strong, rather than taking action only once the body's innate ability has been challenged, and signs and symptoms are present. That's a wellness attitude! The first step is to rid our "self" of toxins, traumas, and negative thoughts on a physical, chemical, and psychological level, and to provide the body with the required ingredients it needs to maintain balance and health. That's body-mind and mind-body healing!

LIFE FORCE & BACK PAIN

THE SACRED GEOMETRY OF THE SPINE

In chiropractic, we begin with the spine, because when we were conceived we were given a brain and a spinal cord first. It is so vital and delicate it had to be encased in an armor of bone. A bony armor if you will.

Our bony armor consists of 26 bones, 23 discs, over 100 joints, hundreds of muscles and thousands of ligaments. It is nature's most powerful and intricate architectural masterpiece. The spine is built for protection and stability, flexibility, locomotion, respiration, and for achieving super-conscious states of being.

Now, the balance between two opposing requirements, such as the need and desire for flexibility, along with the need and desire for protection, means we have to take extreme care of this important instrument. This is because the spine is at the core of everything. Everything is suspended to the spine. It is the infrastructure of the body. It is a support. It has a tendency to collapse if mistreated on a physical, chemical, and/or emotional level. If we break our big toe, it's a bummer. If we break our spine, we're in trouble.

Chiropractic is focused on restoring and maintaining proper spinal motion, alignment, and posture in order to restore and maintain healthy spinal tissues and healthy nerve flow between the body and brain.

The ancient teachers of health and the chiropractors of today understand that healthy spinal bones and joints and free flowing spinal nerve transmission depend on normal spinal motion and alignment. A disruption and decrease in spinal motion and poor posture will result in architectural/structural (bone, joint and tissue) degeneration, along with poor spinal nerve energy flow. The scientific term for this condition is known as a vertebral subluxation.

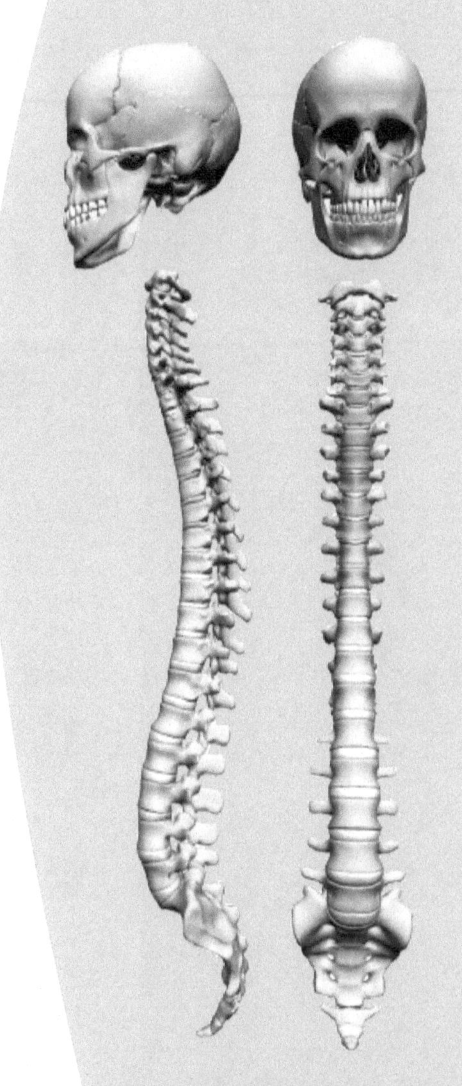

ON SITTING

For thousands of years, yogis sat in a comfortable meditative pose and connected to the energy that permeates the universe. In fact most of the original poses mentioned in the ancient yoga texts are seated ones! As yoga changed over the centuries, thousands of additional poses were identified to prepare the body to be able to sit comfortably in meditation.

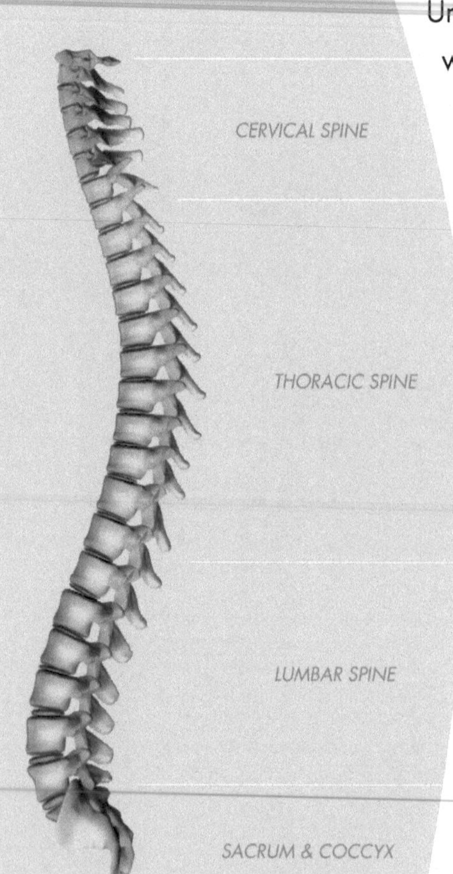

Unfortunately, we now spend on average of 16 hours a day in a seated position, without proper preparation and in chairs. Sitting is to the spine what hard candy is to the teeth! So why is sitting tragic for the spine?

Let's start with some basic spinal anatomy. Let's go back to the womb when we were a fetus. In utero, our spine was C-shaped....one big curve. After leaving the aquatic world, we entered a world where gravity reigns supreme. It took tremendous energy and determination to stand up. First we laid on our stomach and lifted our head up and smiled at the world. Guess what developed? A curve formed in the neck! Our parents probably took pictures of us surfing on our tummy, hands and feet in the air, doing some of our first yoga poses. This position began developing and strengthening our spinal muscles, and created the contours in our spine in preparation for our ascent onto 2 feet to rule the planet...or at least our living room. Then as we learned how to crawl on all fours, another curve formed in the low back. As our mom and dad chased us around the house we were forming a S– shaped curve.

However the average American has lost the S-curve in the spine and in many cases has a reversal of the curve in the neck. Every day, all day, I see people who have lost their natural curves in the neck, quite possibly like you. This puts a tremendous demand on the spine. The spine was built to protect the spinal cord and to act as the core infra-structure for our life! Sitting puts pressure on the nervous system and interferes with the body's ability to communicate with itself and maintain balance and vitality.

The loss of curve happens earlier than one would think. For the comfort and convenience of our parent's active life, many apparatuses have been created to either entertain or contain the baby. Often babies are placed in a vertical contraption, sometimes with wheels. This creates a biomechanical and neurological dilemma. This "walker" allows the baby to propel themselves forward before their spine and pelvis are developed properly for vertical acceleration. By standing upright before the movement is naturally appropriate, the body's balancing/ proprioceptive mechanisms located in the inner ear and upper cervical spine, are tricked into believing that the body can maintain an upright posture. This sets the foundation for unnecessary stress.

Combine this start with the jolts, slips and falls a taken by an adolescent, sliding down the stairs on your behind, the diving headfirst into the couch, the falls off our bicycle, the mandatory extensive sitting in school classrooms, the hours studying at night in the library, and then continuing to sit for hours on end in the work force.

Constant sitting in right-angled chairs, sofas and car seats, often while slouching, does nothing to encourage the natural lordosis in the lumbar spine to continue to maintain its mold. This is how we develop a chronic decrease, and sometimes reversal, of the cervical and lumbar (neck and low back) curves.

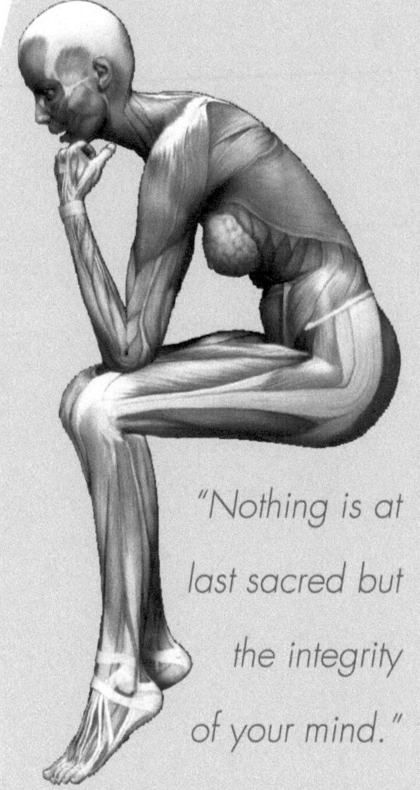

"Nothing is at last sacred but the integrity of your mind."

Ralph Waldo Emerson

You see much of the weight bearing in the spine should take place on your back joints, called facets, and on the back side of the vertebral bodies, this creates a tripod-like structure.

With a loss of curve, weight distribution is removed from the joints and placed upon the discs. Our spinal discs dehydrate, flatten, lacerate and herniate, setting up loss of function and increased pain and suffering. Besides the pain and restriction that develops, you can't sit up tall in meditation.

So now you're asking yourself...what can I do? How about create a new chair with respect to our gravitational demands and our physical design? Until we come up with a new template for sitting on a global level, a good start is to go to a chiropractor to make sure your spine is moving freely, performing optimally, and that spinal degeneration is not present.

Chiropractic is an amazing discipline that helps one keep the bones and joints of the spine moving. Having a freely moveable spine and pelvis, one is able to adapt to the Western industrialized lifestyle, which has sitting as its featured position. Toxic spinal stress created by poorly moving joints activates the stress response and interferes mechanically and metaphysically with the aspirant attempting to sit and meditate.

Another easy proactive step is to begin, or to recommit yourself to a yoga practice. The

ON SITTING *(cont.)*

body is built for movement! And that also means if your job requires you to sit for long periods at a time, invest in a chair that respects your ergonomics, and take frequent movement breaks. You can also do a variety of poses right at your desk. My favorites are the cannonballs, spinal twist, side bends, cervical salutations, standing quadriceps and hamstring stretch.

When sitting in a chair at a desk, or even on your yoga mat, the main self-adjustment you can make is the tilt of the pelvis. As mentioned before in the development of the spine, if the pelvis rotates backward, toward a C-shape, the curve in the low back is reduced leading to stress on the discs. To correct this, finding the front of your sit bones by rotating your pelvis forward to cause the curve to return to its normal shape. This prevents slouching and slumping.

"Affect the unconscious by becoming aware of the conscious."

Dr. Jeremy Brook

Another adjustment you could make is to place a cushion under your sit bones, with a slope downward, to encourage a forward tilt, and to cultivate the return of the lumbar curve.

Continuing with that thread, if you are at a computer desk, put a small pillow behind the small of your back to maintain the lumbar contour. As the great chiropractor Dr. Hugh B. Logan said, "as the sacrum (and pelvis) goes, so goes the spine."

With these minor balancing and positioning modifications we can diminish spinal distortion and degeneration. We'll be able to sit upright and comfortable, and be free to experience the well-being and event bliss that the ancients talk about in their sacred texts.

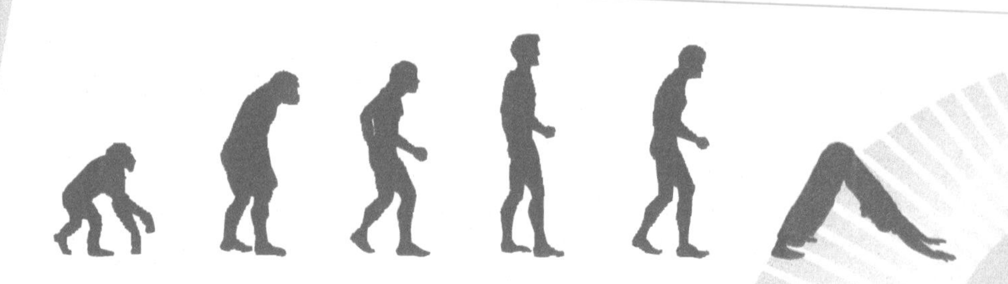

NERVE CHANNELS AND LIFE FORCE

The spine is the means to tap into the inside. It is a fortress of light whose connecting current within gives us the means to access the deeper levels of our self. The ancient disciplines said that this light, life -force, prana or chi, flows through the core or center of the spine via an intricate system of nerves or wires, transmitting life to every cell in the body.

When this "life-force" flows through the body, it activates the intelligence within. When chiropractors use the spinous processes and transverse processes as levers and pulleys to adjust the spine, they can help remove interference that can impede this flow of light within the nervous system.

We now have the science to prove what the ancient Egyptians, Greeks, Hebrews, and yogis spoke about in their sacred texts about the role of the spine and of the nervous system in the preservation of one's health.

This system of nerves is called the nervous system, and is the integrating master of the human ecosystem. It controls and harmonizes our thoughts, feelings, and emotions, as well as coordinates our actions and movements. The nervous system is designed to be a conductor of human electricity. These are sensitive bio-electrical fibers, since, after all, the preferred medium through which electricity travels is a wire.

One Body.

One Mind.

One Spine.

Be One...

NAMES OF ENERGY

The Vital Principle

Have you ever thought about the force that beats your heart and grows your hair and breathes your breath? What IS that? Well, the ideas about what that is are ancient. One of the special components of chiropractic is that it is based on the principle of vitalism.

Vitalism, as defined by the Merriam-Webster dictionary,is:

- *A doctrine that the functions of a living organism are due to a vital principle distinct from biochemical reactions."*
- *A doctrine that the processes of life are not explicable by the laws of physics and chemistry alone and that life is in some part self-determining.*

"What is a man without energy? Nothing - nothing at all."

Mark Twain

Let's begin with a philosophical agreement that there is a Universal Intelligence in all material objects. And inside living beings, we'll call this intelligence... Innate Intelligence. Our Innate Intelligence is activated by an intangible "vital principle" that creates "life" in the body.

This "vital principle" has been a central focus of Homo sapiens since the early days of its existence. Some healers and martial artists have directed their attention on how to increase the flow of this "vital principle" to promote vitality, as well as how to shut off the flow and end life.

According to John White and Stanley Krippner in their book, *Future Science: Life Energies and the Physics of Paranormal Phenomena*, there are at least 97 cultures around the world with a belief in this "vital principle."

Here are a few names it takes worldwide:

Energy
Vital Force
Prana - Indian origin
Chi / Qi - Chinese and Japanese origin
Élan Vital - French origin
Current of Life
Ha - Polynesian origin
Arunquiltha - Australian Aborigine origin
Aché / Axé - Brazilian origin
Boha / Puha - Native American Indian
Vis Medicatrix Naturae - Latin origin

NAMES OF ENERGY *(cont.)*

Megin - Nordic origin
Ruach - Hebrew origin
Ruh - Arabic origin
Human Energy Field - Parapsychological research origin
Light
Somatid - Modern French origin

Some may subscribe to the idea that there is some big, mysterious extra ingredient in all living things, and that dis-ease is the result of some imbalance in the transmission of vital force. Others may look at disease as a result of bad genetics or bad luck.

Whatever our philosophical preference is, creating a lifestyle centered around positive habits gives us the best opportunity to thrive on planet Earth.

After all, we're living on this rock called Earth that's 4. 5 billion years old. At its core, it's about 11,000 degrees hot. It's spinning around the sun at 67,000 m.p.h., on a 584,020,178-mile journey in 365 days, 5 hours, 48 minutes, and 46 seconds.

Innately, we all know that Earth is our mother. Innately we see there is a power organizing and orchestrating life on Earth like a mother nurturing a newborn. When we acknowledge that premise, we are able to trust that Earth heals and rebuilds itself perfectly. Just like our body, Earth needs no interference. No oil spills. No plastic build-ups in the ocean the size of Texas! No pharmaceutical run-off in our rivers. It needs clear air, clean water, and rich soil. These are extremely simple requirements to follow.

Even though we're flying around Earth at 67,000 m.p.h. with molten lava at the core and seasons on the surface, we can trust that the same wisdom running our planet is also running our body. So hold on and get connected to the energy running through you!

"Do you remember the things you were worrying about a year ago? How did they work out? Didn't you waste a lot of fruitless energy on account of most of them? Didn't most of them turn out all right after all?"

Dale Carnegie

WHAT'S A VERTEBRAL SUBLUXATION?

The correction of a vertebral subluxation is the primary goal of a chiropractor. Most people haven't even heard of the term vertebral subluxation, despite the fact that it is a serious obstacle in our expression of health, healing, wellness, and vitality. So what exactly is a vertebral subluxation?

Let us begin with some basic anatomy, physiology, and embryology. When we were conceived we developed a brain and a spinal cord first: these make up our central nervous system. This system, comprised of the brain, spinal cord, nerves, and a dazzling array of neurotransmitters or chemicals by which it communicates, controls, integrates, and harmonizes all the other systems of our ecosystem. It gathers our sensory impressions, coordinates all actions and movements, and is the instrument used in the evolution of one's consciousness. It is the most amazing communication system known to mankind. It is our link to the inner and outer world. It connects us to life.

"You cannot fight darkness, you must turn on light. You cannot fight disease, you must turn on LIFE!"

Arno Burnier, D.C.

Now out from the spinal cord, through holes or channels between the jointed vertebrae, run nerves that carry human electricity, innate force, life-force, light, prana, or chi to every muscle, organ, gland, blood vessel, and cell in the body. Embryology tells us that these nerves are so vital that they must precede the formation of any body part.

Chiropractors are concerned with the relationship between the structure and expression of the human being, specifically the spine and nervous system, and how that relationship may affect one's level of health, creativity, and performance.

There are times in our lives when one or more spinal bones, or vertebrae, lose their normal alignment or motion and cause interference to the spinal cord, which it was designed to protect. The effect is interference and abnormal communication between the brain and body resulting in an altered state of function. This is called a vertebral subluxation.

The vertebral subluxation can arise from causes or imbalances on several levels, due to physical, chemical, emotional, or spiritual stress. These stresses create tension within the nervous system and interfere with the normal flow of human electricity throughout the body. This creates dis-ease within and leads to the expression of thousands of different types of symptoms.

These symptoms are not problems in and of themselves, they are actually signals of the imbalance within. Traumas, toxins, and thoughts are the cause; symptoms are the effects. Chiropractors correct the root cause of the problem by addressing the three T's of the person's lifestyle, rather than treating the effects.

The vertebral subluxation robs the body of focus to think, energy to metabolize, and power to heal. Any interference with the normal action of nerves in carrying human electricity or life-force deranges their functions, and thereby deranges the function of the muscles, organs, or glands to which they travel. The result? An unbalanced body.

This deranged function can only be normalized by having the displacements (subluxations) adjusted, resulting in a free flow of healing energy throughout the body. This is accomplished through the chiropractic adjustment. This free flow of healing energy is felt in every fiber of our being and allows for a most exquisite human experience.

"Look well to the spine for the cause of disease."

Hippocrates

VERTEBRA

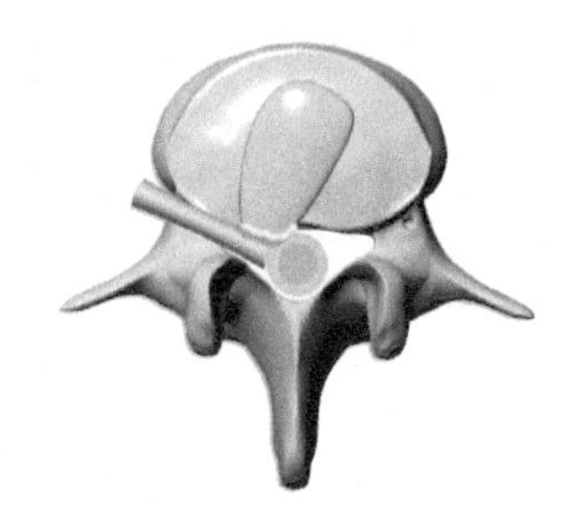

HEALTHY VERTEBRAL ALIGNMENT

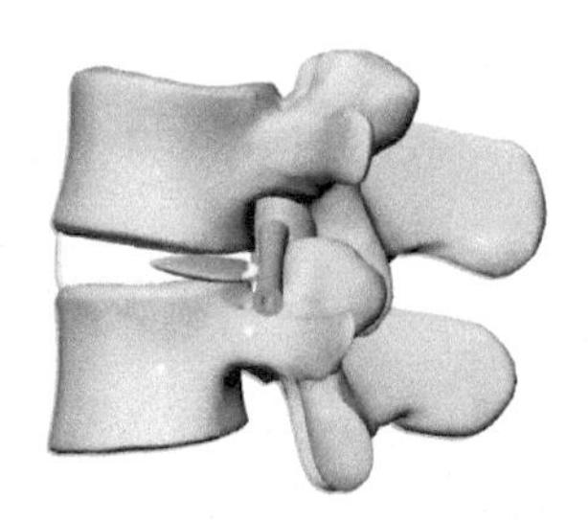

VERTEBRAL SUBLUXATION

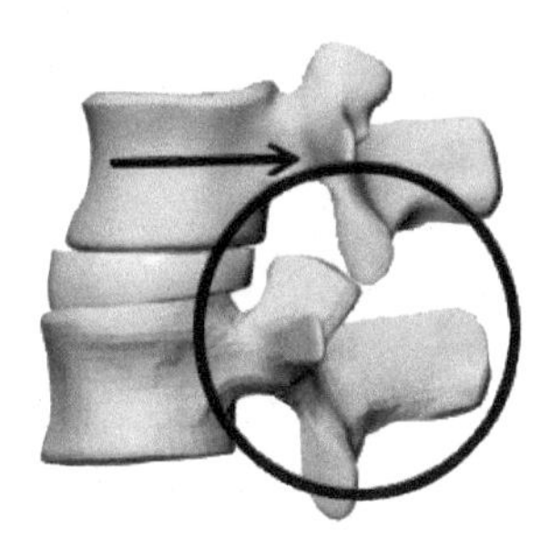

OPTIMAL ALIGNMENT

Any dysfunction of the spine will lead to distortion of the nervous system. That is due to the intimate relationship between structure and function. Structure follows function. Posture will affect neurological function and your expression of life. Distortion in the physical/material system will also cause distortion in the deeper energetic systems. This distortion in the physical system creates a situation where the body is unable to integrate our experience. As a result, tension and stress take hold.

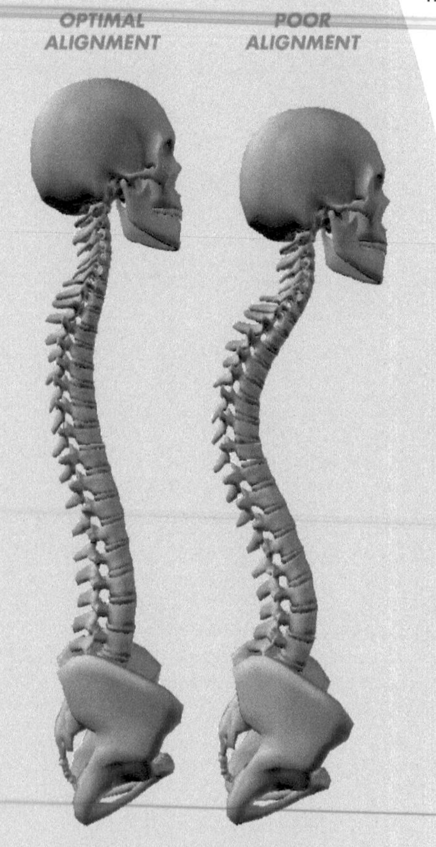

Find your center.

When the spine is stuck, jammed, misaligned, or not moving fluidly, the transmission of energy cannot occur optimally. Optimal nerve flow can be experienced with correct alignment. So what is optimal alignment? It is a state in which the architecture of the body is positioned in such a way that balances gravity, promotes a healthy distribution of weight, encourages full range of motion based on the body's natural design, and allows for the full communication of information and transmission of life-force through the nervous system without interference.

Misalignment is reduced through correct form, proper movement, specific scientific chiropractic adjustments, and intelligent stretching and strengthening. Alignment then leads to powering up the body's energy system. We align our spine so that gravitational forces don't impede the life-force.

The chiropractic lifestyle attempts to maximize the body's ability to integrate life experiences. After all, the main premise of chiropractic is to remove interference from the nervous system to allow the body to express its innate and genetic potential.

The keys to implementing strategies to optimize your health and reduce vertebral subluxation are based on your courage, strength, and fortitude to work toward health, and have the effects of helping to reduce the intensity of your stress response as well as the stressors.

PLANETARY ALIGNMENT ◂

"When Your Inner World Is Aligned, Your Outer World Aligns."

energize it

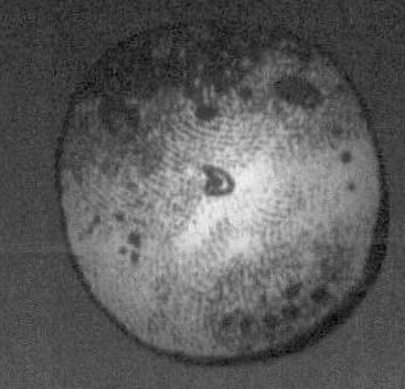

think it

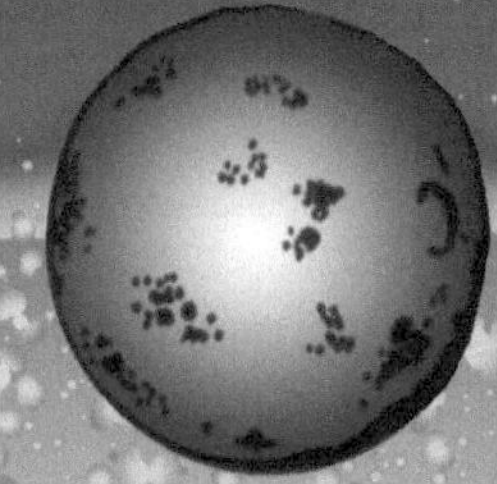

feed it

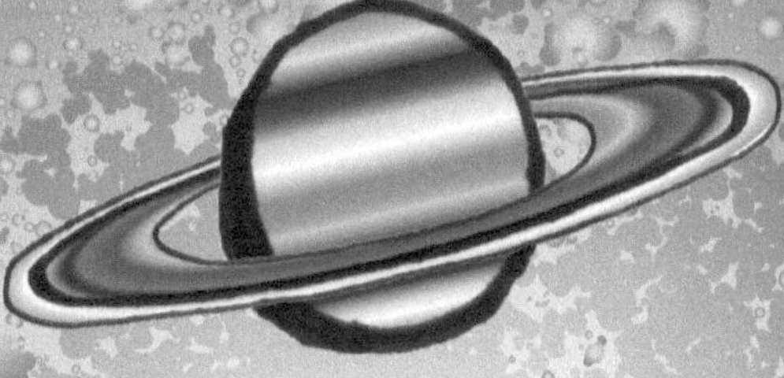

strengthen it

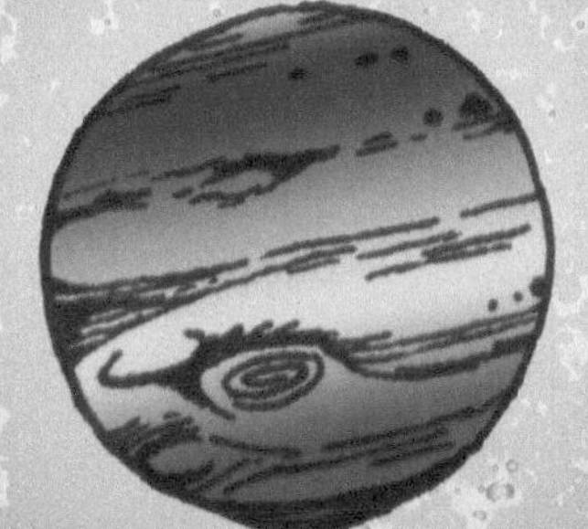

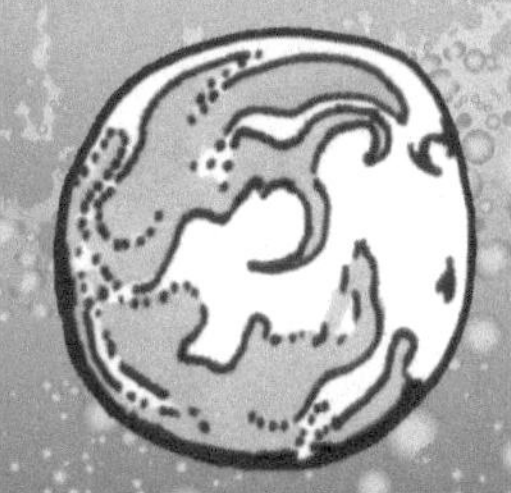

stretch it

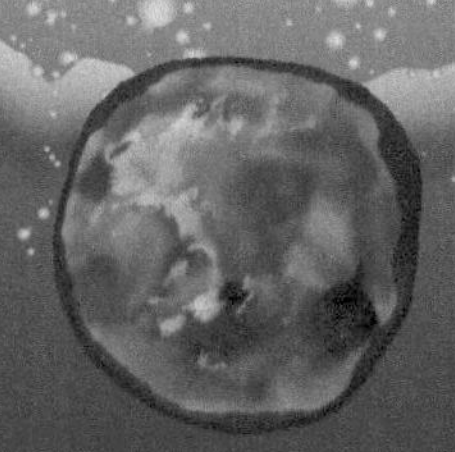

move it

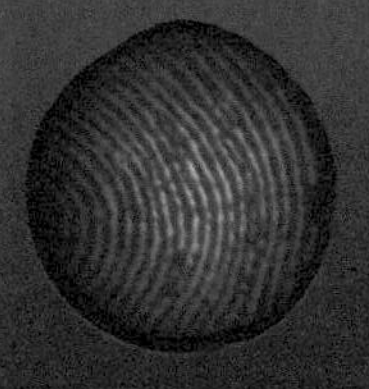

adjust it

MOVEMENT RULES

"The greatest discovery of my generation is that human beings, by changing the inner attitudes of their minds, can change the outer aspects of their lives."

William James

For the first time in history, people are able to scientifically prove what the ancient disciplines taught in their sacred texts about improving concentration and decreasing stress. The key to overall physical and mental health lies in the spine! You may not have even realized that your chiropractic adjustments and yoga practice may be the two most important things you do for the health of your body and mind. A great yogi wrote, "Yoga is the mastery of the activities of the mind-field", or, yoga is about controlling the fluctuations of the mind. But how do we go about this?

Phenomenal research by Jeremy Schmahmann, M.D., has shown how healing movement disciplines, such as chiropractic and yoga, are vital for those striving to achieve total health. His work has shown that movement of the spine stimulates a part of the brain, the cerebellum, responsible for coordinating full body movement, thought, feelings, emotions and organ/immune function.

Specialized receptors, called proprioceptors, located in the joints of the spine, fire when you move the spine, then sending a message to the brain. So what is a proprioceptor? It is a nerve cell found in muscles, tendons, and joint capsules which relays information concerning movements, position and alignment of the body. The highest concentration of proprioceptors in the body is in the spine, with the greatest number gathering in the upper cervical spine.

When a joint moves, the brain wants to know whether or not the movement was healthy. This is huge when you realize that healthy movement of the spine is like atomic energy for your brain. All those sun salutationsd are doing just as much for your mind as they are for your body!

Now, when joints "slam or jam" into each other, proprioceptors don't fire. Rather, nociceptors, or noxious stimulation receptors, get activated and the stress response is triggered. Our fight or flight response can be triggered by the mind, thoughts and perceptions. It can be triggered a woolly mammoth or saber-toothed tiger charging you, and also by a stuck, jammed, or misaligned joint.

Believe it or not, our jammed joints create the same physiological response as being put into a fight or flight situation. Our heart rate quickens, our cardiac output increases, there's a flood of adrenaline, cortisol, and insulin, and a plethora of other reactive responses. That's all from a headstand or upward facing dog gone badly, or hours spent slouched over a computer. Who knew?

Removing irritating or noxious stimulation from our spine with a specific scientific chiropractic adjustment and a dose of smooth, slow and steady movement will decrease our stress response and allow for a positive integration of our thoughts, feelings and emotions.

Yoga evolved from being a secluded meditative practice in which the yogi's asana arsenal consisted of a comfortable sitting pose, to a complicated system of movement and breath. The yogis of old knew that if they could minimize the noxious/nociceptive input into and within the brain, they would be able to decrease the stress response and go deeper into their meditative states. They somehow figured this out without expensive MRIs and CAT scans.

Chiropractic science evolved at a time in history when mankind was most interested in assaulting microorganisms, rather than attempting to strengthen one's innate healing capabilities on the physical, psychological, and spiritual levels. It took pioneers like D.D. Palmer and B.J. Palmer, the founder and developer of chiropractic, as well as modern researchers, to prove that movement of the spine is essential for your health.

Healthy movement can exponentially improve your physiology and psychology just like the great sage told us. That's why chiropractic and yoga are supreme when it comes to exercising our muscles and our mind. It provides the brain with the most essential nutrient for survival...MOVEMENT OF THE SPINE!

With a peaceful mind and strong body, we are able to enjoy life to the fullest and evolve to greater heights. If we can continue to evolve mentally, physically and spiritually, then maybe we can usher in a new revolution based on attaining maximum health, healing and wholeness.....THE WELLNESS REVOLUTION!

"I have to have an adjustment before I go into the ring. I do believe in chiropractic. I found that going to a chiropractor three times a week helps my performance. The majority of boxers go to get that edge."

Evander Holyfield

This essay first appeared in the February, 2009 issue of "LA YOGA Ayurveda and Health"

BRUCE LEE, CHIROPRACTIC & THE REFINEMENT OF THE NERVOUS SYSTEM

Did you know Bruce Lee, in addition to everything else he did, was a writer? It's a fact! He was a true philosopher able to apply specific principles of his martial art to all facets of life. Toward that goal, Lee wrote essays on acting, martial arts, and self-knowledge. He was a modern renaissance man and one of my personal heroes. In fact his book *Bruce Lee's Fighting Method: The Complete Edition* serves as an inspiration for the creation of this manifesto.

"Be like water making its way through cracks. Do not be assertive, but adjust to the object, and you shall find a way around or through it. If nothing within you stays rigid, outward things will disclose themselves."

Bruce Lee

It is not often that we find references to Bruce Lee and chiropractic in the same sentence, but after reading an essay from Lee's classic *The Tao of Jeet Kune Do*, titled "The Importance of Coordination," the connection between the two becomes crystal clear.

In his essay, Lee dives into the different components essential for pure coordination, as well as the importance of refining the nervous system. A master in the martial arts, Lee was highly qualified to write on this topic. In fact, he sounds like a doctor of chiropractic, stressing the importance of possessing a nervous system clear of interference.

Bruce states, "Muscles have no power to guide themselves, but the manner in which they act and consequently, the effectiveness of their performances, depend absolutely on how the nervous system guides them."

Simply put, the nerves deliver a message from the brain, down the cord, out the nerves, to the muscles to give them the power to move. Without proper nerve supply, the muscles are useless. They are, in fact, flesh and meat that become animated when activated by our "inner net" or nervous system. Bruce was a master of his art who knew how to train his nervous system and to harness its power to achieve physical mastery.

In order to achieve optimum command of the physical body, it is essential to understand how the inner wiring is laid out. The inner wiring is responsible for the transmission of human electricity to every muscle, organ, gland, blood vessel, and cell in the body. Without healthy wiring, or nerves, the body becomes weak and lifeless. Thus, one's coordination is affected, resulting in inappropriate reflexes, diminished timing or speed, and imprecise accuracy. That's where chiropractic fits in. Chiropractic is a discipline that concerns itself with the clearing and refinement of the nervous system, and the maintenance of the spinal bones that protect it.

With a clear nervous system, one is able to enjoy a body that is communicating properly within itself. From the brain, the seed and source of the nerve system, down the spinal cord, the most important information superhighway known to mankind, out through the nerves, and to the muscle, flows healing energy. The connection should be a clear one – a clean connection without any interference.

Lee says, " Learning coordination is a matter of training the nervous system and not a question of training muscles. The transition from totally uncoordinated muscular effort to skill is the highest perfection in the process of developing the connections in the nervous system."

If one desires peak physical performance, a sound nerve system is the foundation. The result? A fresh body capable of executing pure power and razor-sharp coordination. So, clear your system – get adjusted!

That's exactly what Lee did with his fighting system. He adjusted his technique, removed the interference and created a complete combat system and philosophy that filtered the impurities from other fighting systems into what he considered to be the bare essentials. Do the same with your health now and you'll be rewarded with the best life has to offer.

"Empty your mind, be formless. Shapeless, like water. If you put water into a cup, it becomes the cup. You put water into a bottle and it becomes the bottle. You put it in a teapot, it becomes the teapot. Now, water can flow, or it can crash. Be water, my friend."

Bruce Lee

THE MOUTH OF GOD: ENTERING THE CAVE OF THE SOUL

"Weaken a bad habit by avoiding everything that occasioned it or stimulated it, without concentrating upon it in your zeal to avoid it. Then divert your mind to some good habit and steadily cultivate it until it becomes a dependable part of you."

Paramahansana Yogananda

The sages of old and the neurologists of today agree that the importance of the upper cervical spine, or the area where your skull sits on the top spinal bone or vertebrae, cannot be overstated. So many of the postures we're striking in yoga class today access this area and have the potential to create incredible breakthroughs in health and insight. As well, they carry a real potential for injury.

A basic, yet thorough, understanding of the anatomy, biomechanics, neurology, and metaphysics of the upper cervical spine is a prerequisite for the yogi to experience increased flexibility, stability, and higher superconscious states. Spinal biomechanical experts Dr. White and Dr. Panjabi describe the upper cervical joint as "...the most complex joints of the axial skeleton, both anatomically and kinematically."

The atlas and axis are two of the nine atypical vertebrae. These two upper cervical vertebrae differ in shape and function from the remainder of the spine. Their design was created to allow for movement, and to provide a base upon which the skull's occiput rests on. These articulations also provide protection for the intimate neurological and vascular structures.

The atlas axis junction is the most freely movable junction in the spine, with respect to rotation (such as looking over your shoulder). This means it can get stuck or compressed with relative ease. Alignment of the bones is imperative, especially since 45-50% of the rotation in the neck comes from the articulation, or movement, of these two bones.

Let's examine some yoga poses:

Take trikonasana (triangle pose), for example. When the yogi looks up and gazes at his top hand, certain biomechanics are necessary to prevent stress and subluxation (misalignment with nerve irritation). A coupling or combining motion needs to take place. When you tilt, or laterally flex, your head to the right, naturally your neck rotates to the same side. So, if you tilt your head to the right and rotate your head to the left, opposite coupling motion takes place. The likelihood of subluxation of the cervical spine is high. You may notice the abnormal biomechanics, or pain, immediately, or perhaps later on in the day.

THE MOUTH OF GOD: ENTERING THE CAVE OF THE SOUL *(cont.)*

So, when practicing any pose that requires you to rotate your head and look upward; such as trikonasana (triangle pose), parsvokonasana or ardha chandrasana, first make sure your head is neutral, gazing straight ahead. Then make a slight head tilt toward the right shoulder, and finally, rotate your head to gaze up at the top hand. This alignment places the spine in the best possible position to move without abnormality and will allow for maximal energy transfer. To feel the difference, tilt your head to the left and rotate your head to the right. Do it slowly – it may be much harder!

* See Neck Handout (pg. 80) for further illustrations

The yogis of old innately knew how to move their bodies with great care. They somehow psychically downloaded information on the neuroanatomy and physiology of the upper cervical region. They discovered that the upper cervical spine represents a transitional area where the brain and spinal cord make love, a portal for the awakening of insight and awareness.

With skillful and intelligent movement of the spine you can look up to the stars and dive inward into an ocean of peace and calm. Should you get stuck, call your local chiropractor!

"Misdirected life force is the activity in disease process. Disease has no energy save what it borrows from the life of the organism. It is by adjusting the life force that healing must be brought about, and it is the sun as transformer and distributor of primal spiritual energy that must be utilized in this process, for life and the sun are so intimately connected."

"IS YOGA SAFE?"

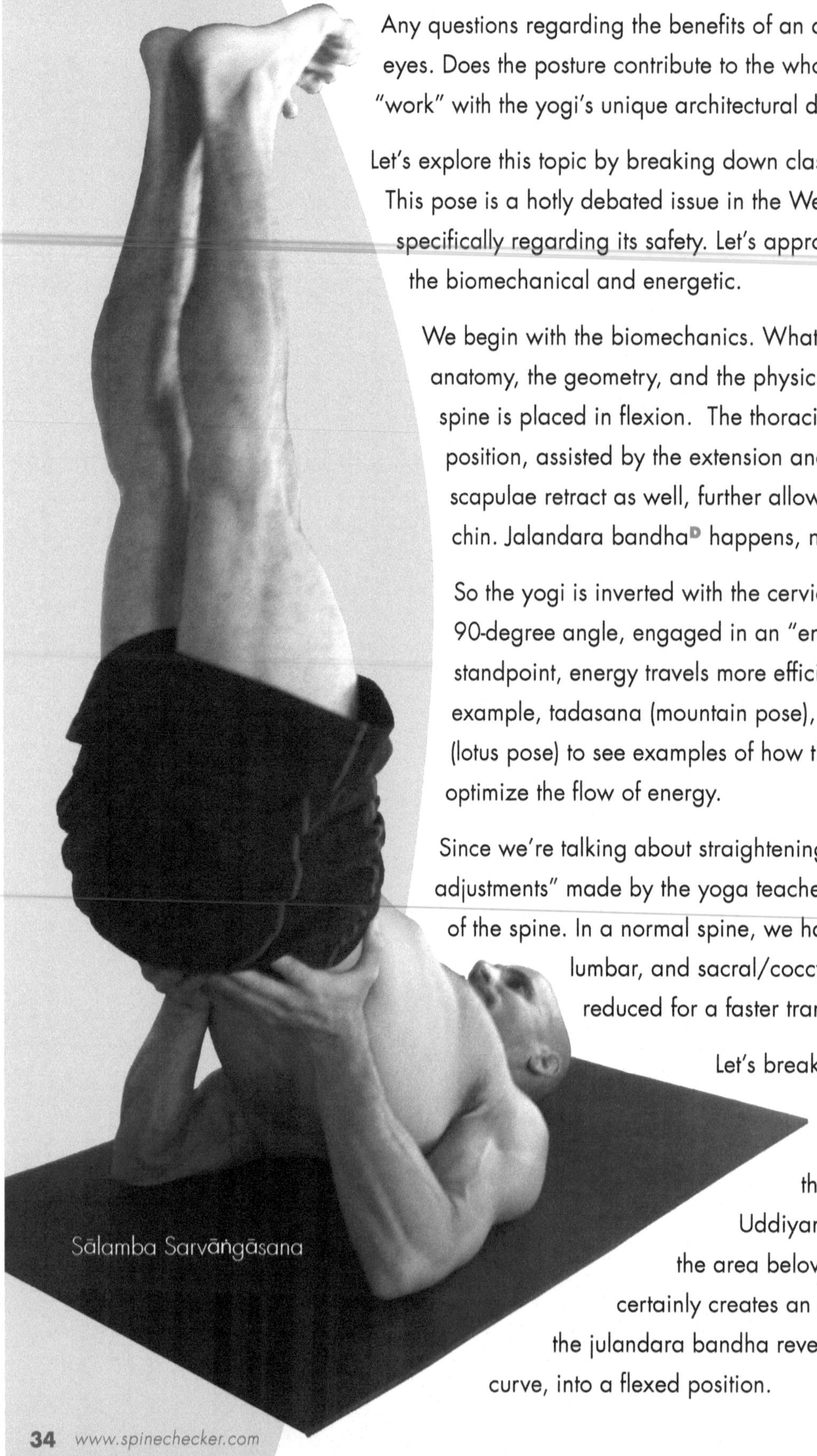

Any questions regarding the benefits of an asana should be seen through holistic eyes. Does the posture contribute to the whole of the being? Does this posture "work" with the yogi's unique architectural design? Does it create vitality or toxicity?

Let's explore this topic by breaking down classic sarvangasana, or shoulderstand. This pose is a hotly debated issue in the Western health care community, specifically regarding its safety. Let's approach it from two different perspectives: the biomechanical and energetic.

We begin with the biomechanics. What is the design of the pose... the anatomy, the geometry, and the physics? From the ground up, the cervical spine is placed in flexion. The thoracic spine is placed in a slightly extended position, assisted by the extension and external rotation of the humerus. The scapulae retract as well, further allowing the sternum to draw closer to the chin. Jalandara bandha[D] happens, naturally and ideally, if all goes well.

So the yogi is inverted with the cervical spine and thoracic spine in a 90-degree angle, engaged in an "energetic lock." From an energetic standpoint, energy travels more efficiently through a straight spine. Take for example, tadasana (mountain pose), dandasana (staff pose), or padmasana (lotus pose) to see examples of how the yogi "straightens" his/her spine to optimize the flow of energy.

Since we're talking about straightening the spine, some "corrective adjustments" made by the yoga teacher are aimed at minimizing the curves of the spine. In a normal spine, we have four curves: cervical, thoracic, lumbar, and sacral/coccygeal. In shoulderstand these curves are reduced for a faster transmission of energy.

Let's break it down energetically. Activating mula bandha[D] causes the lumbar spine to straighten, or flatten, as the coccyx moves toward the pubis. Uddiyana bandha[D] will add to this by drawing the area below the belly-button in and up. This certainly creates an awesome lift. Then the application of the julandara bandha reverses the last of the curves, the cervical curve, into a flexed position.

Sālamba Sarvāṅgāsana

From an energetic point of view, these actions can generate a profound experience and, if done repeatedly, can bring about a shift in consciousness.

So, back to the mat. The yogi is inverted with the weight of his entire body supported, ideally, on the outer shoulder, triceps, and elbows. The problem I have, chiropractically speaking, with this awesome pose, is that today's yogi sits at a desk for six, eight, or even twelve hours a day, comes home, collapses into his/her down sofa, and then goes to sleep on their stomach. I am generalizing, but you get my point.

This isn't the yogi we read about from the days of yore who practiced yoga for six hours a day, meditated for three, read from the sacred texts for several hours, and then fell asleep on a hard bed made of straw.

Today's yogi has the same spirit of the yogis of old, but the problem is the curve in his neck is reversed, and possibly degenerated. On top of that, the average person has been in one or more car accidents, and this compounds the stresses in the spine. The forward head or reverse curve position puts an incredible amount of stress on the discs, the facet joints, and most importantly, the nerves. Then, in addition to an architecturally challenged neck, the yogi goes upside-down and rests the weight of his upper body straight above a very delicate part of the spine, the cervicothoracic junction.

One of our main concerns has to do with the integrity of the cervical discs. The discs in your neck are not able to handle stress very well when weight is being loaded upon them. In fact, the flexed position with compression will cause the nucleus pulposus, the inner part of the disc, to bulge outward and backward toward the outside of the disc, called the annulus fibrosis. The bulge of the annulus can cause irritation to the spinal nerve or even the spinal cord itself, potentially resulting in the radiation of pain into the shoulders, arms, and hands. When that happens, one's asana practice, and one's life for that

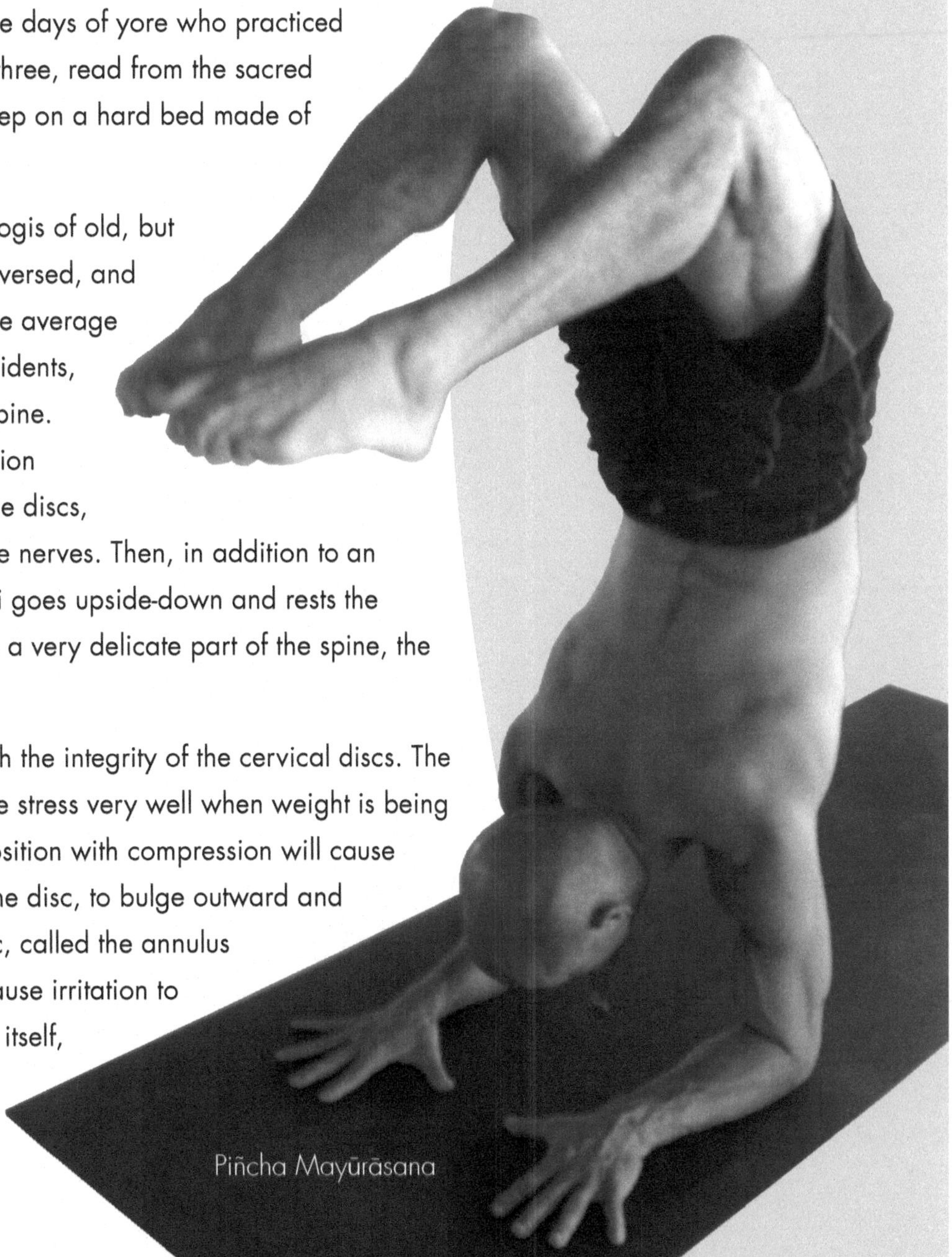

Piñcha Mayūrāsana

"IS YOGA SAFE?" *(cont.)*

matter, becomes challenging.

The bottom line? The disc has its greatest ability to become damaged with the neck in a flexed position and loaded with weight. Great to remember if you are sparring with a jujitsu opponent, not so great if you are trying to bathe that area in free-flowing prana.

So if you have degeneration in your neck, or a loss of a cervical curve, a modified shoulderstand may be appropriate. In this version, the weight of your lower body rests on your hands, like a kick-stand. You'll form three angles in this position rather than two. This will surely take the pressure off anyone's neck.

Another option is to use blankets to help elevate the shoulders and take pressure off the neck.

"You're only as young as your spine is flexible."

Yogi Bhajan

These are suggestions to make your asana practice safer and more energy efficient. My recommendations are based on creating stability and ease within the body. I do not subscribe to any style of yoga which attempts to fit the person to the exact picture of pose. The yogi should customize the asana to match his/her mind-body-type. That is true yoga! Too many injuries occur as a result of people doing asanas that aren't congruent with their architectural design.

That is why self study of your body is vital. Know your limitations...know your strengths...and then move slowly and skillfully with them in mind. With impeccable movement you are able to harness the energy and wisdom that the sages of old wrote about, and can still experience the intensity of the practice without injury.

This essay first appeared in the July/August, 2007 issue of "LA YOGA Ayurveda and Health"

CELLULAR VITALITY

REINCARNATION

After gestating for 280 days a human being is born and thrust into this world. During this period of time a bewildering sequence of events transpires under our eyes, or rather, in the belly of the expectant mother. A new life form is created and shaped by an innate, or inborn, intelligence that contains the perfect recipe for transformation and growth. It's in every fiber of our being, breaking us down and rebuilding us again. That's right.... every cell in the body dies and is reborn anew.

"Health is a state of complete harmony of the body, mind and spirit. When one is free from physical disabilities and mental distractions, the gates of the soul open."

B.K.S. Iyengar

If you don't believe in reincarnation, just look under a microscope and you'll see a universe of cells sprouting, dividing, multiplying, dying, sprouting, dividing, multiplying, and dying. Cells transform from healthy to dis-eased, as well as from dis-eased to healthy. And that's how our body works until our last breath where there is no more division, only cell death.... which according to the mystics, frees the soul from its physical confines.

Take into consideration that our body is being recreated every second. Our body's ability to rebuild itself around good alignment depends on the lifestyle choices we make. Our choices/stresses/actions - physically, emotionally, mentally, and chemically - will either build us up, constructively or down, destructively.

Our body is so intelligent it does whatever it needs to do to survive and reproduce. It takes what we give it and builds us from those materials, whether it's from our mental thought forms, our raw kale salad, our daily yoga practice, or our specific chiropractic adjustments.

We need to look within and ask ourselves, "What do we need to do to rebuild our 'self' stronger, wiser, and even more intuitive, so that we can live in a sustained state of bliss and health?" Bliss and health will be achieved when we create healthy cells for a sustained period of time by making intelligent lifestyle choices. Intelligent lifestyle choices decrease accelerated cellular aging.

When we get down to the sub-atomic level of our cells, we find that the physical structures disappear and all we are left with is pure energy. Energy and matter are one! We are energy bodies! To maintain high voltage energy levels we need the trillions of cells diving, multiplying, and repairing at an optimal level. And our lifestyle choices shape our energy and cellular reincarnation!

HEALING AT THE SPEED OF LIGHT

Twentieth century research purports that nerve impulses can travel as fast as 225 - 250 miles an hour! Not quite the speed of light, which travels at 186,000 miles per second, but still extremely fast.

From our days in high school biology, we learned that nerve impulses travel through the nervous system to our organs, glands, muscles, and blood vessels. Our nervous system resembles the ultimate transportation system…a superhighway!

Our nervous system boasts an intricate design that relies on a logical series of events to trigger an appropriate body response. Without this system, we could not exist. Our information superhighway needs to be free of interference to enable efficient travel. Nothing is worse than going on a road trip only to find out that you are stuck in bumper to bumper traffic and all the exit lanes are closed. We want to travel the open road with no obstacles.

That is why healing disciplines of the East together with holistic practitioners of the West focus on maintaining open lines of communication within the body. If there is interference along the pathway, messages are slowed or altered, resulting in dis-ease and sickness.

Holistic practitioners and adherents of holistic disciplines recognize that interference can occur on several levels: structural, chemical, and mental, any of which alter our body's ability to expand into it its own electromagnetic energy field.

"Only recently have scientists and physicians begun to appreciate the key role which mechanical forces play in biological control at the molecular and cellular levels."

Donald Ingber, M.D., PhD.

One major source of interference can be found in the brain. This mysterious three-pound organ of fat and water is unique to all creation in its design. The brain can have a misalignment in its protecting cranial joints, called sutures, interfering with its ability to control, originate, integrate and harmonize information. The brain's bony armor, the skull, is made up of twenty-two sheet-like plates that are interconnected through approximately sixty razor sharp teeth, called sutures. That's right.... The implication of this is that the skull can misalign, resulting in interference to the rhythmic expansion and contraction occurring at the sutures.

Misalignments to the spine can interfere with both spinal cord and spinal nerve functions, effectively interrupting healing impulses which would otherwise travel to the brain. When this happens, our internal experience of our bodies, as well as our external experience of the world at large is altered accordingly. Miscommunication within our

HEALING AT THE SPEED OF LIGHT *(cont.)*

communication/energy/electrical system causes us to age at an accelerated rate leading to dis-ease and sickness. This is astounding to absorb when you realize that our body's cellular age may be only around 25 years old even if your actual birth-age is 40. Within the human body, the normal aging process is regulated by a mechanism called **apoptosis**, or the pre-programmed life span of a cell. For example, the densest of all cells, the bone cell, can last up to 25-30 years before the cell dies! Our muscles push/pull and carry us around for about 15 years. Other cells, like our white blood cells, can last from a couple hours to a couple days. Sperm cells: around two to three days. Same with the stomach lining cells which live for about two days. The oxygen-carrying red blood cells last longer, and live for roughly 120 days.

"The best methods are those which help the life energy to resume its inner work of healing."

Paramahansa Yogananda

There are a number of factors that determine the length of the life of each cell. Traumas and toxins and unhealthy lifestyle can certainly cause a rapid decline in the health of our cells. On a positive note, when we provide our body with its basic requirements, the cell's apoptosis rate can be slowed down considerably.

Here's how: humans replace worn-out cells through cell division. In 1965, a brilliant professor at University of California at San Francisco, Dr. Leonard Hayflick, discovered there is a certain number of times a human cell will divide before it stops dividing, at which point in time it dies. A cell usually dies after 52 divisions. This is called the Hayflick Limit.

Here's a little more cell biology for you. Each time a cell divides to replicate, the DNA unwraps and the information in the DNA is copied. On the end of the DNA strand lies a structure called a telomere. Telomeres are like shoelaces. Telomeres protect chromosomes and prevent them from fusing into rings or binding with other strands of DNA. Now, each time a piece of the DNA is unwrapped and copied through division, it takes a piece of the telomere, or end of the shoe lace with it. The telomeres lose a little bit of length each time this happens. When the telomere is reduced to a certain length, the cell dies. Therefore, one of the components in aging is how often the cells divide and the length of the corresponding telomeres.

If we can somehow give our cells the best environment possible to ensure that they don't divide at an accelerated rate, we can age beautifully, naturally and gracefully. It is more intelligent to take care of the body before abnormalities are felt in the tissues or seen in laboratory tests. It's an active approach to life that requires us to make responsible choices.

REPAIR AND REGENERATION

When we experience stress and trauma, the intelligence of our body begins immediately to repair the damage. This requires a healthy flow of communication across our nervous system to oversee and organize the prepping and cleaning up of the injured area so new growth can begin.

New growth will be incomplete if the body is unable to detect where the injury has occurred and where to start the repair job. That's why holistic doctors emphasize removing interference from the body's inherent ability to heal itself, called above-down-inside-out healing, so that it can orchestrate an effective healing response. An effective healing response involves a repair and a remodeling phase.

The repair phase, the prepping and cleaning, takes time. It's not an overnight job. Sometimes it can take 6 weeks or longer to clean up and repair a wound...a wound that develops due to traumas, toxins, or negative thoughts. This phase is similar to the "prep-phase," when you tear down an old room and build a new one. During the initial phase, the debris gets removed, the new wall get spackled, and old walls get broken down. It doesn't look pretty. Inside the body, the repair phase looks like an organized mess. That's because the walls aren't painted and there's still no furniture. If the nervous system communicates effectively with all of its workers and has all of the appropriate building blocks, the prepping and cleaning up is accomplished quickly.

Give a man a fish and you feed him for a day; teach a man to fish and you feed him for a lifetime.

Maimonides

Once the body repairs the damage, the body transitions into a detailed and organized restructuring phase which can take up to 36 months! This is called the remodeling phase. In this phase, the body smoothes out the patchy unfinished business started in the initial repair phase. The rough edges are diminished and the tissues become more functional. Once our body has repaired and remodeled itself, the healing of the stressed-out site becomes stabilized.

The rate and efficiency with which our body will repair, remodel and stabilize itself is determined by our strength of adaptability, the amount of stresses we experience, past physical, chemical and mental damage, and the amount of nerve energy flow coursing through our body without congestion and stagnation.

Body-mind training gives our body the best opportunity for repairing, remodeling and stabilizing itself from the inside out! Without interference, our body can express itself to its maximum potential, and reach new heights of wellness and performance.

LIKE SANDS THROUGH THE HOURGLASS, SO ARE THE DAYS OF OUR LIVES...

One morning while I was walking barefoot on Venice Beach, a thot-flash (chiropractic slang for a download of awareness and insight) came to me. As my feet sunk into the beach beneath me, I thought of an hourglass filled with sand. The hourglass represents our health and the sand represents the traumas, toxins, and negative thoughts that accumulate over the years. When we turn the hourglass upside down, the base layer of sand represents the oldest physical, emotional, and chemical stresses, and the sand on the top represents most recent.

"As it took time for the condition ... to change from health to a maximum degree of abnormality ... it takes time to retrace ... back to health."

B.J. Palmer

When we embark on a path of healing, both new and old issues rise to the surface. That's why dormant injury or trauma may be re-experienced in the form of symptoms even though it happened years or even decades before. This phenomenon of healing is called "retracing" and is based on the work of Dr. Herring. He said that healing happens in five directions: above, downwards, within, outwards, center to periphery, from more important to less important organs, and in the chronologically reverse order of disease development.

As the body moves toward wellness, it must first retrace the trajectory of the deviation. It's like an archeological dig within your hourglass, uncovering trauma treasures. During this archeological dig, the body may experience and express symptoms associated with past traumas, toxins, and negative beliefs that we store in different parts of our body and access through the nervous system. Even though these symptoms may be uncomfortable, they are not to be judged as negative. If traced and embraced with care they may lead to transformational breakthroughs on a body-mind level.

For some, retracing can be intense, whereas for others, the taste of old residue is no big deal. Since we all have different body-mind constitutions, we tend to retrace differently. One element we have in common is that our bodies become more efficient as they filter out old debris.

Like sands through the hourglass, so are the days of retracing.

HUMAN BIOLOGICAL CLOCK

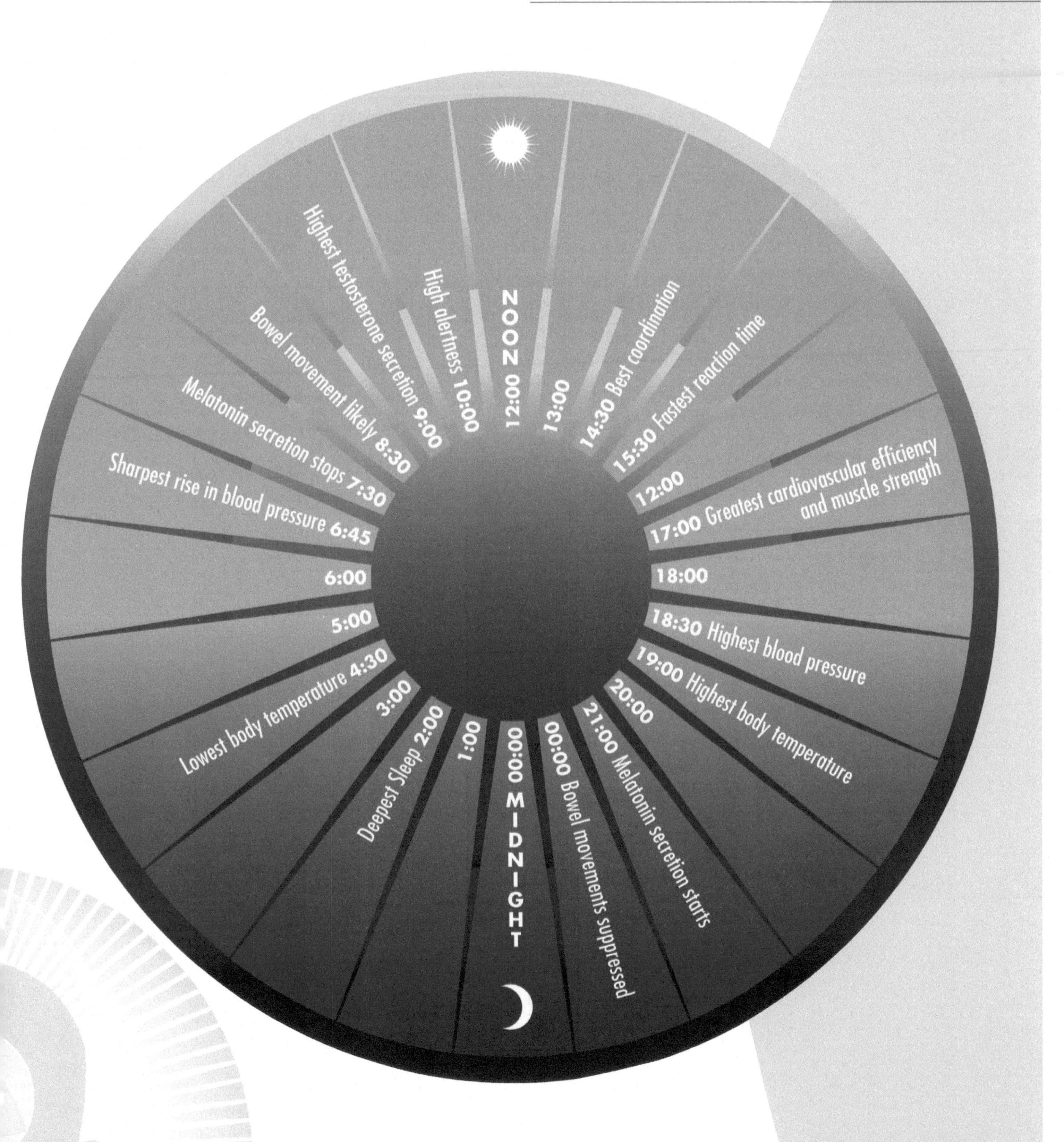

This chart was derived from an original at http://en.wikipedia.org/wiki/Circadian_rhythm

CHILL OUT

When *Homo sapiens* stood up on two feet a million years ago a dramatic event took place. By standing up vertically, instead of walking on all fours, mankind shifted the orientation of his spine and allowed for energy to flow more efficiently. According to a new theory published in the July 2007 issue of The Journal for the Proceedings of the National Academy of Sciences," humans walking on two legs consume only a quarter of the energy that chimpanzees use while "knuckle-walking" on all fours. However, we continually deplete this energetic advantage by activating our stress response unnecessarily and, many times, chronically.

Our stress response is one of the most important programs installed by a universal intelligence into the animals of the Earth. The stress response enables us to sense danger and was designed to do one thing: keep us alive. For primitive man, life on the plains could be rough. Back then we had great animals like saber-toothed cats, giant ground sloths, mastodons, and mammoths that could create a big problem for us if we were caught off guard.

"Tension is who you think you should be. Relaxation is who you are."

Chinese Proverb

Good thing we have a component of the nervous system that works immediately to resolve any perceived or real threat. In 1936 a Hungarian doctor, Hans Selye, discovered in the laboratory what the ancients had discovered in the worlds' highest mountain caves, the physiology of stress. Selye conceptualized the physiology of stress as having two components: a set of responses which he called the "General Adaptation Syndrome," and the development of a pathological state from chronic, ongoing, unrelieved stress.

The General Adaptation Syndrome, or G.A.S., can be broken down into three stages:

Stage 1: Alarm

Stage 2: Resistance

Stage 3: Exhaustion

In stage 1, Alarm, our nervous system detects a stressor, in the form of a trauma, toxin, or thought, which sounds the alarm bells, whistles, and sirens. During this stage, the body undergoes a cascade of identifiable reactions, releasing chemicals and hormones, such as adrenaline and cortisol, to deal with the dangerous threat or stressor. Just think of the legendary comic book superhero, the Incredible Hulk. When scientist Dr. Bruce Banner is physically, emotionally, or chemically threatened, his alarm is triggered and he transforms into the Hulk.

First, Dr. Banner's nervous system detects the stressor, which sends a message to the famous hypothalamus-pituitary-adrenal gland axis. Immediately, the Hulk's heart rate goes up, blood is shunted from the skin and organs and is sent to the muscles. That's usually when the Hulk starts tearing through his expensive designer clothes. The next step involves getting more energy from the energy reserves so Hulk can do his smashing thing!

Here's a more detailed account of what happens:

- Acceleration of heart and lung action
- Constriction of blood vessels in many parts of the body
- Liberation of nutrients for muscular action
- Dilation of blood vessels to and within muscles
- Inhibition of stomach and intestinal action
- General effect on the sphincters of the body
- Inhibition of lacrimal gland (responsible for tear production) and salivation
- Dilation of pupils
- Relaxation of bladder
- Inhibition of erection
- Auditory Exclusion (loss of hearing)
- Tunnel Vision (loss of peripheral vision)

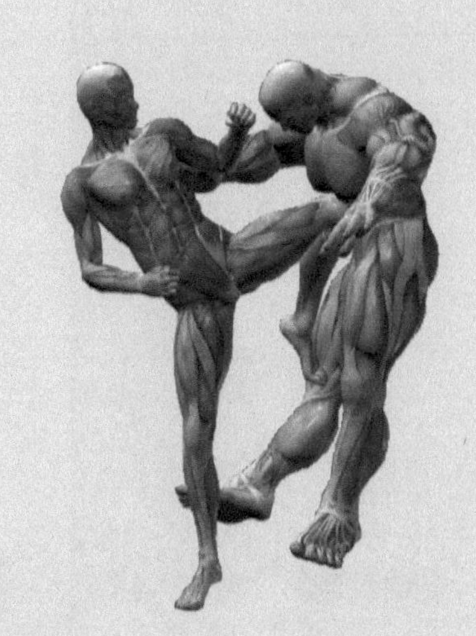

(Guyton M.D., Hall Ph.D.. Textbooks of Medical Physiology, 9th Ed. W.B Saunders Co. 1996, p. 779)

All of these effects are normal and necessary to survive a life- threatening situation and get us to safety. But they aren't healthy for long periods of time. If the stressor persists, the body enters into the second stage, the **resistance stage**, where we try to adapt to the ongoing stressors. However, the body is unable to maintain resistance indefinitely, and, as a result, the body-mind suffers as its resources are gradually depleted.

Once the body's resources have been taxed and depleted like a ruthless dictator ruling over his helpless citizens, the body is unable to maintain normal healthy function. This is where the body enters the third stage, **exhaustion**, where chronic dis-ease becomes the norm.

Negative effects of a chronic stress response manifest in all systems of the body and

CHILL OUT *(cont.)*

mind, resulting in depressed immunity, decreased energy, decreased muscular performance, decreased sex drive, abnormal digestion, increased risk of cardiovascular accident, obesity, and diabetes to name a few. Just imagine how the Hulk would feel if he went on a rampage for hours, days, weeks, and months in your neighborhood. He would be exhausted!

We could take a page out of the Ice Age, the Medieval Age, and even the Modern Age, and the stress response would be exactly the same. That's right, there would be no change in the basic physiological reaction. When we joined communities about 10,000 years ago and created prototype cities, technically our stress response – which is to fight or flight - should have decreased because of our newly found safety from the harsh environmental conditions. That wasn't the case. While the stress response was designed for small, brief, acute situations, it has unfortunately become a daily and regular occurrence in our lives, wreaking havoc on our health.

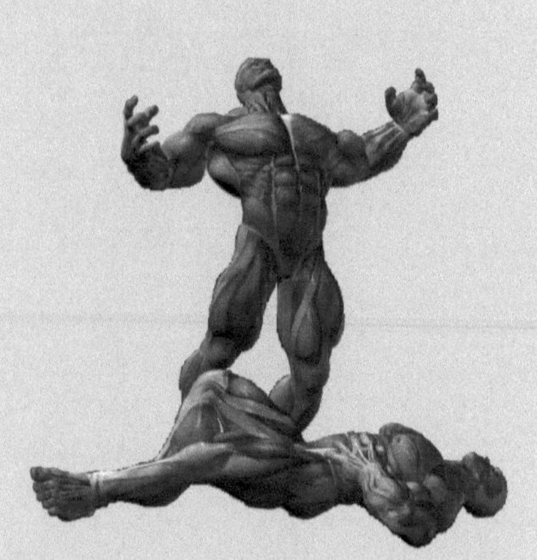

We're not battling saber-tooth predators anymore. Today we battle traffic, overbearing people, obnoxious news reports, junk food, unpaid bills, unemployment, overly medicated sick grandparents and poorly designed furniture, to name a few, all of which trigger the stress response! Thankfully we have the ability to tap into our innate ability to control the reflexive activation of the stress response.

Some people are better than others at their ability to control their stress, unlike the Hulk. Yogis and martial artists have proven in scientific demonstrations their skill at controlling their stress response and physiology through moving and breathing techniques. Their feats are bewildering and illustrate the amazing potential lying dormant within.

Some basic steps we can take to improve our physiology and decrease the activation of the stress response include chiropractic adjustments, yoga, breathing techniques, and a contemplative meditation practice. We don't have to be prisoners of stress. Through disciplined effort we can achieve our destiny as warriors of health and wholeness!

MUSIC OF THE SPINE

Did you know the origin of chiropractic is based on tone and vibratory waves in the body? When spinal bones lose their "tone, or pitch," as a result of traumas, toxins, and negative thoughts, the result is what chiropractors call a vertebral subluxation, or a movement deficiency syndrome TM (a term coined by Dr. James Chestnut) that affects not just the fluid movement of the spine, but also the health of our thoughts, feelings, emotions, and immunity. Locating and correcting vertebral subluxation allows our body to find its natural baseline pattern. Unfortunately, it may take years for us to tune our spine and body its natural rhythm!

The human body is very similar to a finely tuned musical instrument. Every cell in the body emits a certain frequency. When our body is in alignment, the music is beautiful. When the spine is misaligned the tone is "off" and the music sounds distorted.

The quieter you become, the more you can hear.

Ram Das

When enough cells are vibrating at the right frequency, we experience resonance, or a community of cells vibrating at the same rate and rhythm. All of the cells "tune in" to the same vibration and produce one healthy sound. For example, if we hold something vibrating at another object's resonant frequency very close to the object, the second one will begin to vibrate at its resonant frequency without physical contact. Strike a tuning fork and hold it a couple of inches away from another tuning fork of the same frequency, the second one will begin to vibrate even without being struck. So cool! Hold it next to a tuning fork of any other frequency and nothing will happen. To give another example... we're in a yoga class. In the beginning we chant the scared mantra AUM. Some yogis are in key and some are off. But by the middle portion of the chant, magically most are in tune. Health is the same way! Our body loves being in alignment and in tune. The greater the number of healthy cells, the greater the expression of health will be. When our vertebrae are misaligned, the sound is jumbled and distorted, and the music is painful to the ears.

Through extensive research, pioneers in sound and vibration are able to locate the specific frequency of our spinal bones. That's right! They can actually be tuned. Each vertebrae of the spine differs in age, size, shape, and density, and has its own natural frequency of vibration. My mentor, chiropractic master Dr. Arno Burnier, taught me to feel for the vibration of the vertebrae to tap into the harmonics that lie within the spine and feel if it is vibrating at an altered rate.

MUSIC OF THE SPINE *(cont.)*

Dr. June Leslie Wieder's research in sound healing and vibrational therapy using tuning forks has given us frequencies for each vertebrae. She states, in her book *Song of the Spine*, that, "these frequencies are not absolute. ....In the future, more exact data will likely be obtained from the use of a tunable electronic instrument in place of a simple tuning fork." Dr. Wieder is currently working with engineers to create such a device that more accurately tunes our spine. So in the meantime...to keep our instrument in great form and sounding beautiful...get aligned and get moving!

Frequencies of the Vertebrae:

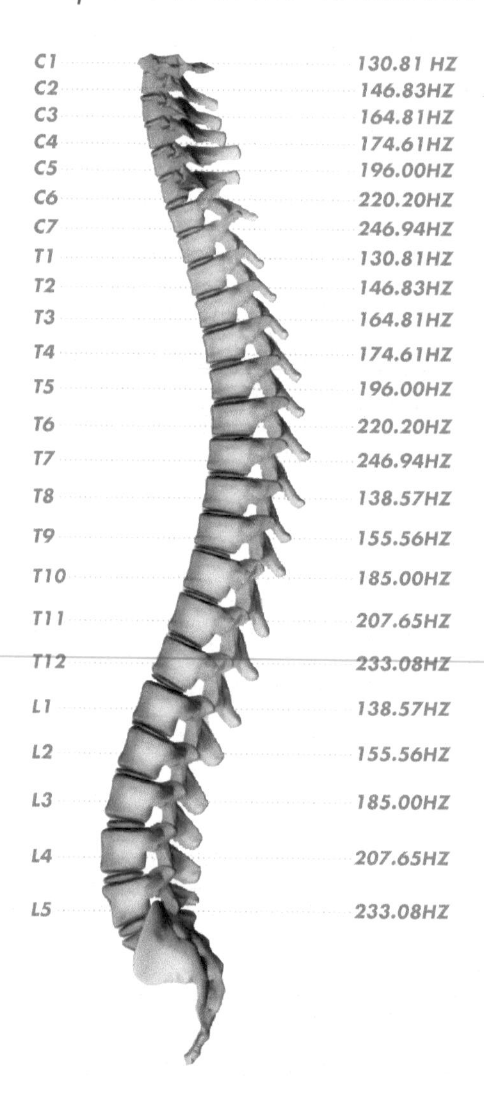

Dr. June Leslie Wieder

from "Song of the Spine"

INCREASED VITALITY

Chiropractic was introduced to mankind in 1895 as a discipline to remove nerve interference, thereby allowing the body to sprout, divide, multiply, and die at a normal frequency... a frequency of healthy cells producing healthy tone/ vibes/ rhythm. With healthy tone and vibration, the body ages gracefully.

To give an analogy, visualize Caesar Milan, the Dog Whisperer. Caesar rehabilitates traumatized dogs, as well as their owners, by teaching them how to organize their energy and balance their tone. Think of a leash connected to the dog's collar. Caesar teaches that the owner's energy is transmitted through the leash to the dog. Now, when the owner is relaxed, the tone or tension of the leash is relaxed, and the dog stays calm and relaxed. If the owner is stressed and grips the leash tightly, the tone or tension of the leash becomes tight, and the dog becomes stressed and anxious. If the owner is lazy and fails to hold the leash, the tone or tension of the leash becomes too loose, and the dog runs away.

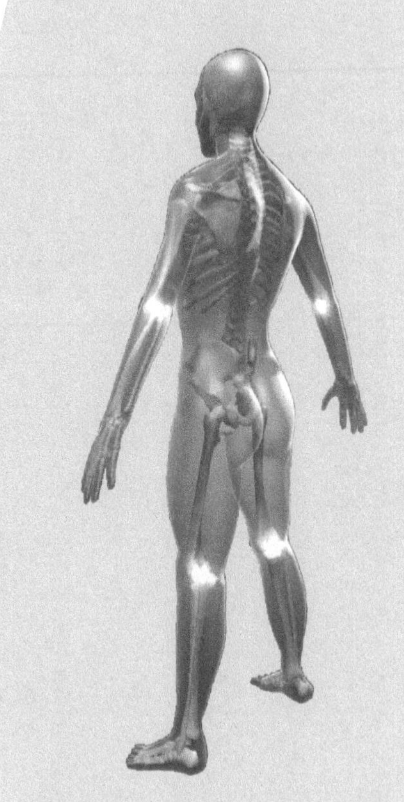

Our nerves behave just like a leash...they transmit energy. But instead of a dog at the end of a leash, we have muscles, organs, glands, and blood vessels. Normal nerve tone produces a state of ease within the body. Stressed nerves produce hard muscles, organs, glands, and blood vessels. Slack nerves produce limp and lazy muscles, organs, glands and blood vessels. Think of your retirement savings disappearing...ouch...your nerves become tense. Drink a can of soda and you'll feel your nerves become excited. If you go snowboarding and land hard on your sacrum, you'll feel your nerves sharply. Imagine yourself at a time in your life when you were at your strongest and happiest, your nerves will relax. End of story. The key lies in developing lifestyle strategies that create balanced healthy tone, which results in increased vitality!

Increased vitality is our natural baseline state! People we know are misaligned on multiple levels and then make resolutions and dedications to reclaim their health once a year. That's fine, but maintaining an attitude of vitality makes more sense than repeatedly having to reclaim it. It takes more energy to have to generate the will power to "get healthy again." Just do it! (I think I've heard someone say that before).

Chiropractic, like Caesar Milan, strives to maintain healthy energy flow. So the next time you walk your dog, check your energy, and see if your dog behaves differently. Or how about with your lover, your children, or your parents!? Then apply the same lesson to your body and your nerves. With a healthy nerve energy flow your body is able to move naturally through the rhythm of life.

FORCE FIELD

On June 24, 2008, my 88- year old grandfather suffered a major stroke that left him bedridden. Interestingly enough, at that exact time I began to feel a disconnection with the left side of my arm, hand, and body. It was as though I was feeling the effects of his stroke. Thankfully, he has since recovered. He sleeps a lot, smiles like a newborn baby, and has moments when he is conscious and present, although the physical act of speaking remains a challenge. When he does talk, words come out primarily in his native tongue, Hungarian, of which I only understand: "I love you;" "thank you;" "Yes;" "no;" and a handful of bad words he taught me. Still, we share a non-spoken connection wherein we can just hold hands and look at each other and feel pure love.

"The Force is what gives a Jedi his power. It's an energy field created by all living things. It surrounds us and penetrates us. It binds the galaxy together."

Obi-Wan Kenobi,
Jedi Master

Once in a while I will experience the tension in my body and assume that my grandpa is having a T.I.A., or a minor stroke. I'll call my grandma to ask how he is doing, and she'll say, "He is sleeping a lot more, but he is the same." This leads me to believe that my energy, or electromagnetic field, is connected to his, and when he experiences a change in his field, I get a sense of it. Clearly, I'm sharpening my extrasensory skills.

Current research shows that an electromagnetic field surrounds our bodies. This electromagnetic field receives input from our mental thought patterns. Depending on our mental thoughts, our energy field can be positively affected, which nourishes the body, or negatively impacted, which stresses the body. Basically, our thoughts affect our energy field, which in turn affects the body.

So it is essential to make sure that the mental thought forms in our mind's eye are of a positive vibration. We, the leaders of the new paradigm, choose high vibing, empowering thoughts over weak ones that would otherwise seek to disempower us and wreak havoc on our bodies, mind and spirit. We must choose to stand guard like a warrior for automatic false thoughts that have no real basis in the real world. Breathing and concentration techniques followed by affirmations are effective ways to flood the mind with healing thought forms, which are then absorbed into the body like food.

By sending healing thought forms and affirmations into our electromagnetic force field, we turn off the stress response and activate the relaxation response, which allows our body to receive a healthy flow of positive energy. This enables our body-mind to reach its true life potential, while expanding the truly infinite powers of our consciousness.

Think for a moment of your body basking under the sun. Feel how the sun nourishes and revitalizes the body. Your thoughts behave the same way. They can burn you or keep you warm.

Our energy field appears to be the link between the mind and body. I like to think that the mind and body are one. When we acknowledge this concept as a collective entity we may enter a reservoir of untapped energy.

There is so much about the human body that we have yet to explore. For hundreds of years, the geocentric model was the predominant scientific model that placed Earth at the center of the universe. Soon this model was found to be erroneous. It wasn't until the 16th century that the model we understand now was identified in Western thought, when mathematician and astronomer, Copernicus, presented a mathematical model of a solar system that placed the sun at the center of the universe. Those who supported this model were considered heretics and were burned at the stake. Ouch!

Gregg Braden, Rupert Sheldrake, and other scientists have already PROVEN that there is a morphogenic field surrounding the planet and that we live in a holographic universe and no one is suggesting burning them at the proverbial stake.

I am excited about the opportunity to break old boundaries and attitudes about the human body and be a pioneer in a new wave of consciousness, connectedness, health and healing. Talk about a wellness revolution!

"When cells band together in creating multicellular communities, they follow the 'collective voice' of the organism, even if that voice dictates self-destructive behavior. Our physiology and behavior patterns conform to the 'truths' of the central voice, be they constructive or destructive beliefs."

Bruce Lipton, Ph.D., in The Biology of Belief

OLD SCHOOL PHILOSOPHY

OLD SCHOOL CHIROPRACTIC PHILOSOPHY

You may be asking yourself, "What is old school chiropractic philosophy doing here?" Actually, the founders of chiropractic were way ahead of their time.

Since its founding in 1895, chiropractic has been a hot topic of controversy and criticism with mainstream medicine because of its vitalistic beliefs. In fact these beliefs landed many chiropractors in jail in the early part of the 1900's! Fortunately, now it is not uncommon to see medical doctors, and even surgeons, getting adjusted before they head off to see their patients.

These medical doctors may not "believe" in the transmission of life-force, but they'll take their kids to the chiropractor to get their spine adjusted because when they do, their asthma goes away. Or maybe they'll take their elderly parent to the chiropractor to get that small bone at the top of their neck adjusted, because when it is misaligned their blood pressure goes through the roof. Or maybe they'll go in themselves for an adjustment before a four hour surgery, because if they don't they'll wake up in the morning unable to walk and they don't want to have to take pain pills and muscle relaxers.

So I hope you enjoy a teaser trailer of old school chiropractic philosophy! For more cutting edge philosophy check out Dr. Simon Senzon's books, "The Spiritual Writings of B.J. Palmer" and "The Secret History of Chiropractic: D.D. Palmer's Spiritual Writings, Vol. 2."

ANCIENT CHIROPRACTIC

Adjustments of the spine go way back. The first evidence of spinal manipulation was depicted in cave drawings discovered in France dating back to 17,500 B.C. Battling some primitive bear could surely have thrown out someone's back. Or just imagine how a caveman's neck would feel after sleeping on a cold rocky floor. Ouch! A caveman manipulation of some sort would surely be required!

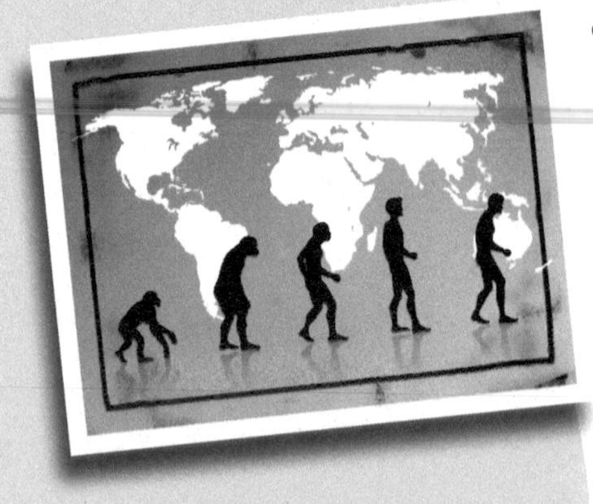

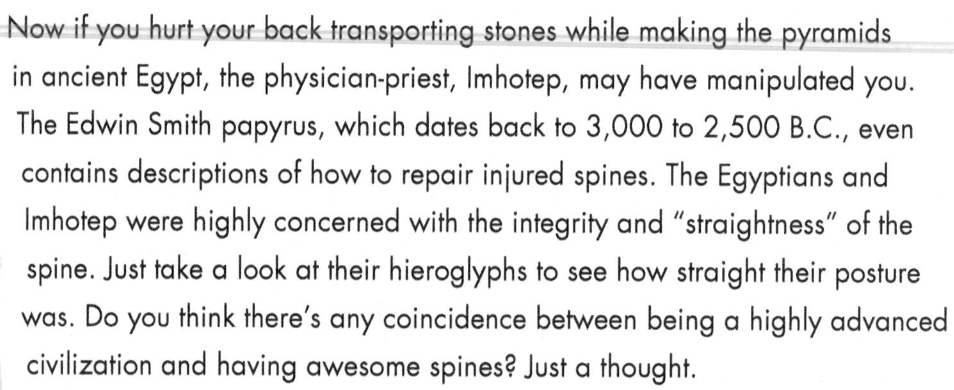

Now if you hurt your back transporting stones while making the pyramids in ancient Egypt, the physician-priest, Imhotep, may have manipulated you. The Edwin Smith papyrus, which dates back to 3,000 to 2,500 B.C., even contains descriptions of how to repair injured spines. The Egyptians and Imhotep were highly concerned with the integrity and "straightness" of the spine. Just take a look at their hieroglyphs to see how straight their posture was. Do you think there's any coincidence between being a highly advanced civilization and having awesome spines? Just a thought.

Although the Chinese were best known for their needles, they were performing spinal adjustments in 2,700 B.C. according to the Kung Fou Document.

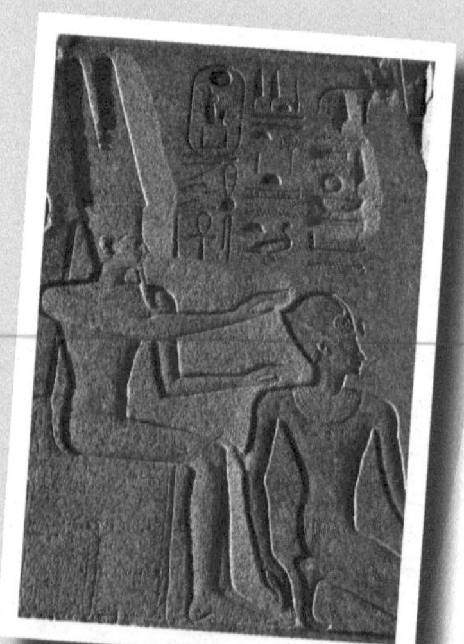

Just over the Pacific Ocean, in America, there are tales of a powerful spinal manipulator, called "Dances with Spine," who danced on injured spines to bring them back to life. Actually I made that up, but the Sioux, Winnebago, and Creek Indians related spinal manipulation to the healing of the body. And down the road in Central America, the Mayan and Aztec Indians also routinely utilized spinal manipulation in their healing arts before the Spanish wiped out their culture, medicine, and religion.

The ancient origins of chiropractic can be traced back to ancient Greece to the time of Hippocrates, Galen, and Asclepius. Hippocrates, a drug-free physician credited with over 70 books dedicated to the healing arts, was a big fan of spinal manipulation. Around 500 B.C. Hippocrates wrote two best sellers called Manipulation and Importance of Good Health and another work called Setting Joints by Leverage. The major premise of the books… "Get knowledge of the spine, for this is the requisite for many diseases."

The work of the Greeks were carried over to Rome, as Galen, known as the "Prince of Physicians" during 2nd century A.D., taught the importance of proper spinal alignment. He was known for the saying, "Look to the nervous system as the key to maximum health." Interestingly, in 195 B.C., he was crowned with the title "Prince of Physicians" after manipulating the neck of Eudemus, renowned Roman scholar, restoring function to his once paralyzed hand.

The gradual infiltration of the Roman world by a wave of Conan-like barbarians in the Dark Ages was followed by a period of stagnation in the sciences and manipulation of the spine went out of style. Talk about a subluxation! The union of the mind and body was shattered amongst the collective consciousness. The care of the physical body rested in the hands of the physician and the care of the mind and spirit under control by the priests. It would be in a few hundred years before mind and body could be reunited, and care for the whole person would be reestablished. You could thank the chiropractors for that!

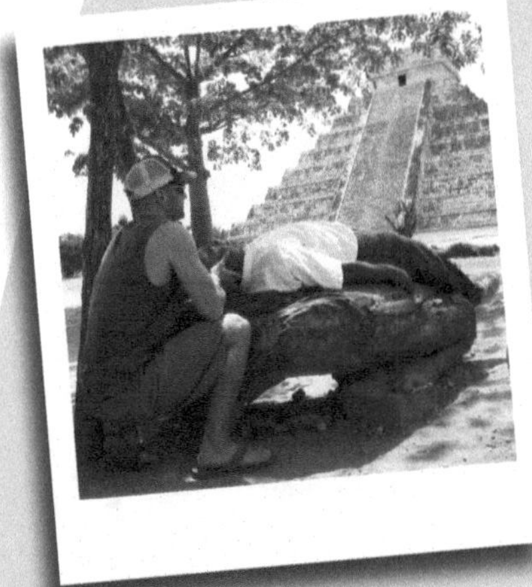

This is me giving a Mayan an adjustment at Chitchen-Itza

But all was not lost. Some of the old techniques were handed down from generation to generation and there are many recorded cases of European "bone-setters" performing amazing acts of healing. During this time manipulation was handed down through families of "bonesetters." In France a bonesetter was called a rebouteux, in Germany a knocheneinrichter, in Spain an algebrista, and in Denmark as kloge folk. *(FJH Wilson, Chiropractic in Europe: An Illustrated History, 2007, page 13)*. The famous Sweet Family practiced bone setting in New England in the mid 19th Century.

Overall, the 19th century in Europe and America was a time of turmoil, controversy, as well as incredible breakthroughs in the realm of health and philosophy. Crude manipulation of various forms continued in many cultures all over the world until 1874 when Andrew Taylor Still, the founder of Osteopathy, brought manipulation back into vogue. Years later in 1895, D.D. Palmer, the discoverer of modern day chiropractic, found a "vertebra racked from its normal position" in his deaf janitor's spine, and decided to adjust it. Out of this episode, the most advanced style of spinal adjustments was born. Crude traction, bone-setting and general manipulation gave way to specific scientific chiropractic adjustments.

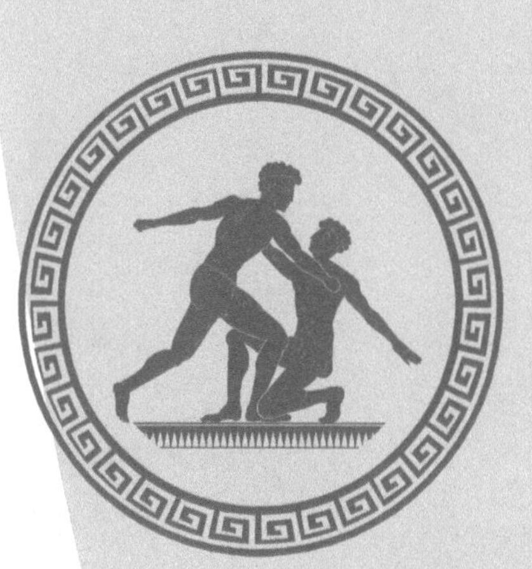

The mid late 20th century has been a tremendous advancement for humankind. As incredible techniques have sprouted up within the chiropractic profession, helping to propel our physical, emotional, mental, and spiritual evolution to untapped heights. I can't wait to see what the future holds!

THE BIG IDEA

by B.J. Palmer, Developer of Chiropractic

A slip on a snowy sidewalk, in winter, that is a small thing. It happens to millions.
A fall from a ladder, in summer, is a small thing. It happens to millions.
A slip or fall produces a subluxation. The subluxation is a small thing.
The subluxation produces pressure on the nerve. That pressure is a small thing.
The pressure cuts off the flow of mental impulses. That decreased flowing is a small thing.
That decreased flowing produces a dis-eased body and brain. That is a BIG thing to that man.

Multiply that sick man by a thousand, and you control that physical and mental welfare of a city.
Multiply that man by a million, and you shape the physical and mental destiny of a State.
Multiply that man by one hundred and thirty million and you can forecast and prophesy the physical and mental status of a nation.
So the slip or fall, the subluxation, pressure, flow of mental impulses, and dis-ease are big enough to control the thoughts and actions of a nation.

This man is given an adjustment. The adjustment is a small thing.
The adjustment replaces the subluxation. That is a small thing.
The adjusted subluxation releases the pressure upon the nerves. That is a small thing.
The released pressure restores health to a man. That is a big thing to that man.

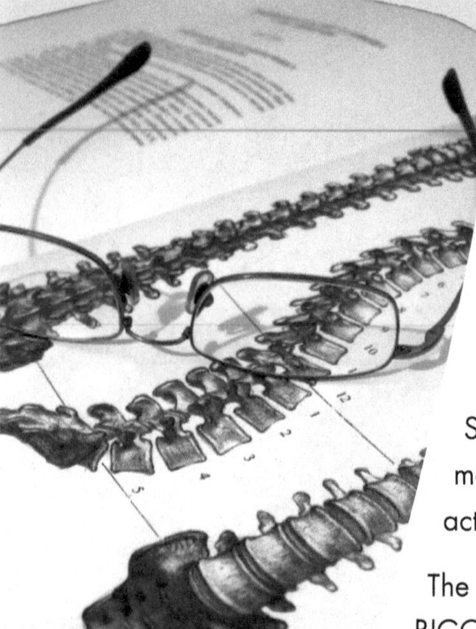

Multiply that well man by a thousand and you step up the physical and mental welfare of a city.
Multiply that well man by a million, and you increase the efficiency of a State.
Multiply that well man by one hundred and thirty million, and you have produced a healthy, wealthy, and better race for prosperity.

SO the adjustment of the subluxation, to release pressure upon nerves, to restore mental impulse flow, to restore health, is big enough to rebuild the thoughts and actions of the world.

The idea that knows the cause, that can correct the cause of dis-ease, is one of the BIGGEST ideas known.
Without it nations fall; with it nations rise.

The idea is the biggest one I know of.

THE TRUTH

By B.J. Palmer

"We Chiropractors work with the subtle substance of the soul. We release the imprisoned impulse – the tiny rivulet of force – that emanates from the mind and flows over the nerves to cells and stirs them into life. We deal with the majestic power that transforms common food into living, loving clay; that robes the earth with beauty, and hues and scents the flowers with the glory of the air."

"In the dim, dark, distant long ago when the sun first bowed to the morning star, this power spoke and there was life; it quickened the slime of the sea and dust of the earth and drove the cell to union with its fellows in countless living forms. Through eons of time, it finned the fish and winged the bird and fanged the beast. Endlessly it worked, evolving its forms until it produced the crowning glory of them all. With tireless energy it blows the bubble of each individual life and then silently, relentlessly dissolves the form, and absorbs the spirit into itself again."

"And yet you ask 'Can Chiropractic cure appendicitis or the flu?' Have you more faith in a spoonful of medicine than in the power that animates the living world?"

THE 33 CHIROPRACTIC PRINCIPLES

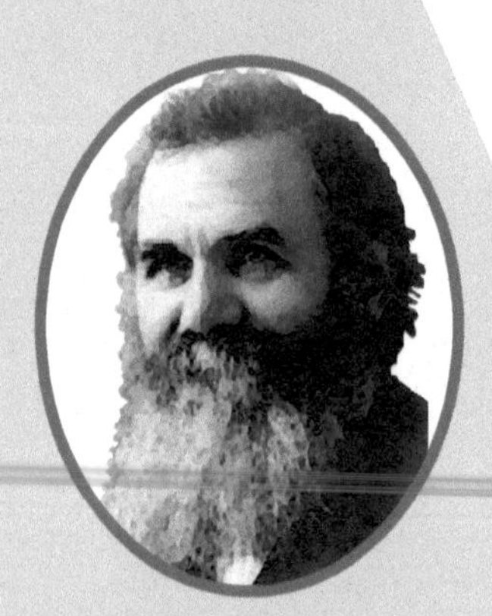

*Doctor D.D. Palmer (father)
Discoverer and Founder of
Chiropractic*

In 1927, Dr. Ralph W. Stephenson, in his book, *"Chiropractic Textbook"*, consolidated the philosophy of chiropractic into thirty-three concise principles...appropriately called the Thirty-Three Principles. These principles provided an intellectual, philosophical, scientific, and artistic foundation for the bourgeoning chiropractic profession, and represented the essential dimensions of chiropractic's unique approach to health, healing, and optimal life expression.

The Thirty-Three Principles provide the missing link between mind and matter, force and intelligence, energy and life. They help explain abnormalities in anatomy and physiology and how to restore and refine health and banish dis-ease. Some principles are carried over from the great wisdom teachings, while others are completely unique to our time.

The Thirty-Three Principles are based on the premise that the human body is composed of trillions of cells that are interconnected in a self-healing, self-regulating ecosystem. Chiropractors recognize that the body requires no intervention and no interference with its innate abilities of self-expression and self repair. This premise is no longer considered alternative, as recognized names including Drs. Andrew Weil, Deepak Chopra, Bruce Lipton, Candice Pert, and Joseph Mercola base the core premise of their teachings on concepts that chiropractors have been teaching since 1895! Because of these doctors, the chiropractic message is breaking through the medical hierarchy and is slowly becoming integrated into the new energy medicine paradigm. Thanks to past geniuses, like Albert Einstein, and advances in technology, these principles are proving to be true and relevant in our daily lives.

"Have you more faith in a knife or a spoonful of medicine than in the power that animates the living world?"

Dr. B. J. Palmer

As you read through the Thirty-Three Principles, you may detect a basic organization. They're categorized into three general natural categories: **universal principles, biological principles,** and **chiropractic principles**. Each principle dives holistically into the nature of organization in the universe, the relationship between intelligence and matter in living things, and lastly, chiropractic's laser sharp focus on the relationship between the nervous system and the spinal column.

Excerpt from Chiropractic Textbook:

"Some of the principles are basic, upon which others are founded or derived as going from the general to the specific; some are down to a part of the whole thing. These specific principles are, of course, derived principles. They are not limited to any given number. A fundamental principle of Chiropractic is a statement of the quality or actions of intelligence in matter, which will include any and all circumstances that may arise in study."

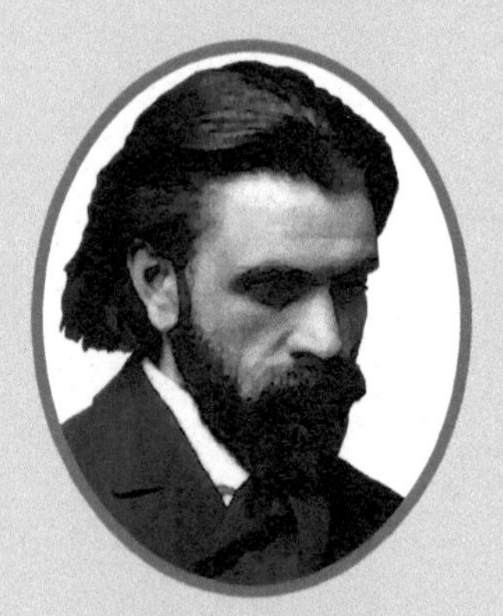

*Doctor B. J. Palmer (son)
Developer of Chiropractic*

THE 33 CHIROPRACTIC PRINCIPLES *(cont.)*

1. The Major Premise - A Universal Intelligence is in all matter and continually gives to it all its properties and actions, thus maintaining it in existence.

2. The Chiropractic Meaning of Life - The expression of this intelligence through matter is the Chiropractic meaning of life.

3. The Union of Intelligence and Matter - Life is necessarily the union of intelligence and matter.

4. The Triune of Life - Life is a trinity having three necessary united factors, namely: Intelligence, Force and Matter.

5. The Perfection of the Triune - In order to have 100% Life, there must be 100% Intelligence, 100% Force, 100% Matter.

6. The Principle of Time - There is no process that does not require time.

7. The Amount of Intelligence in Matter - The amount of intelligence for any given amount of matter is 100%, and is always proportional to its requirements.

8. The Function of Intelligence - The function of intelligence is to create force.

9. The Amount of Force Created by Intelligence - The amount of force created by intelligence is always 100%.

10. The Function of Force - The function of force is to unite intelligence and matter.

11. The Character of Universal Forces - The forces of Universal Intelligence are manifested by physical laws; are unswerving and unadapted, and have no solicitude for the structures in which they work.

12. Interference with Transmission of Universal Forces - There can be interference with transmission of universal forces.

13. The Function of Matter - The function of matter is to express force.

14. Universal Life - Force is manifested by motion in matter; all matter has motion, therefore there is universal life in all matter.

15. No Motion without the Effort of Force - Matter can have no motion without the application of force by intelligence.

16. Intelligence in both Organic and Inorganic Matter - Universal Intelligence gives force to both organic and inorganic matter.

17. Cause and Effect - Every effect has a cause and every cause has effects.

18. Evidence of Life - The signs of life are evidence of the intelligence of life.

19. Organic Matter - The material of the body of a living thing is organized matter.

20. Innate Intelligence - A living thing has an inborn intelligence within its body, called Innate Intelligence.

21. The Mission of Innate Intelligence - The mission of Innate Intelligence is to maintain the

"Watch your thoughts; they become words.

Watch your words; they become actions.

Watch your actions; they become habits.

Watch your habits; they become character.

Watch your character; for it becomes your destiny."

Upanishads

THE 33 CHIROPRACTIC PRINCIPLES *(cont.)*

material of the body of a living thing in active organization.

22. The Amount of Innate intelligence - There is 100% of Innate Intelligence in every living thing, the requisite amount, proportional to its organization.

23. The Function of Innate Intelligence - The function of Innate Intelligence is to adapt universal forces and matter for use in the body, so that all parts of the body will have coordinated action for mutual benefit.

24. The Limits of Adaptation - Innate Intelligence adapts forces and matter for the body as long as it can do so without breaking a universal law, or Innate Intelligence is limited by the limitations of matter.

25. The Character of Innate Forces - The forces of Innate Intelligence never injure or destroy the structures in which they work.

26. Comparison of Universal and Innate Forces - In order to carry on the universal cycle of life, Universal forces are destructive, and Innate forces constructive, as regards structural matter.

"Dwell as near as possible to the channel in which your life flows."

Henry David Thoreau

27. The Normality of Innate Intelligence - Innate Intelligence is always normal and its function is always normal.

28. The Conductors of Innate Forces - The forces of Innate Intelligence operate through or over the nervous system in animal bodies.

29. Interference with Transmission of Innate Forces - There can be interference with the transmission of Innate forces.

30. The Causes of Dis-ease - Interference with the transmission of Innate forces causes in coordination of disease.

31. Subluxations - Interference with transmission in the body is always directly or indirectly due to subluxations in the spinal column.

32. The Principle of Coordination - Coordination is the principle of harmonious action of all the parts of an organism, in fulfilling their offices and purposes.

33. The Law of Demand and Supply - The Law of Demand and Supply is existent in the body in its ideal state; wherein the clearing house, is the brain, Innate the virtuous banker, brain cells clerks, and nerve cells messengers.

EAT, SLEEP, & BE HAPPY

THE SCIENCE OF WELLNESS

Wellness is a term generally used to mean a healthy balance of the mind-body and spirit that results in an overall feeling of well-being. The premise of wellness is that we can live a long, fulfilling, and active life as long as we provide our body with its basic requirements and needs, or as Dr. Chestnut would say: "purity and sufficiency." It's sad to see our parents, grandparents, or loved ones, taking a tray full of drugs to treat ten different symptoms because they neglected to take care of themselves early on.

"Scientists were rated as great heretics by the church, but they were truly religious men because of their faith in the orderliness of the universe."

Albert Einstein

One of the first realizations we need to make is that humans are animals with highly developed brains. Biologically we're no different. Our bodies behave in the same manner as other animals do to poor diet and exercise regimes. Give a great ape a fast food hamburger, French fries, and a diet-cola and see if that massive and beautiful animal gets stronger or gets sicker. If we remove the great ape from its mountain habitat and place it in a barren sterile enclosed cage it gets sick. Return it to the jungle where it can eat, roam and exercise the way it was created, and it becomes healthy again. We need to return to the jungle!

The human animal diet and physical fitness have changed dramatically over the last century and not all of it for the better. There has been a new medical movement to place blame on our poor health and chronic disease patterns on genetics. But we can't blame our genetics if we don't eat the food that our body was designed to eat, or if we don't move enough. When we shifted our hunter and gatherer lifestyle to farming lifestyle, our bodies had to adpat. Thankfully they do it. But our new lifestyle, which is difficient in movement and toxic with sugar and starches, has taken a toll on our health.

It is unfortunate that billions of dollars have been spent cracking the code of the human genome. Twenty-five thousand genes in the human body were found, however cell biologists say there are over 100,000 genes they have yet to identify. That's like saying you identified all of the countries of the world but left out Europe, Australia and Asia. A list like that cannot be considered complete. According to these biologists, we have a lot more discovering to do in the genetic realm. Adding insult to injury, our genetic code has barely changed in the last 40,000 years so we can't really blame our genes for making us prone to cancer, heart disease, obesity, diabetes and so on.

We are just slow to adapt to the new health challenges we have imposed upon our genetic makeup since our hunter and gatherer days. In time, we may evolve to process refined sugars and starches efficiently. In time we may learn how to process junk food. But until we develop mutations, we will express symptoms and must contend with the consequences of a lifestyle that is inappropriate for our current physiological design. Type 2, or adult onset diabetes, may be one of the consequences of our inappropriate diet and lifestyle that has arrived. We are not evolved enough to live a chronic sedentary life, eat poor food, and have negative thoughts. We have to behave like our ancestors of 10,000 years B.C. So that means if our parents or grandparents had heart disease, our fate isn't sealed because of their genes. Our lifestyle choices reduce the chance of repeating our family's history of poor health.

According to Drs. Bruce Lipton, author of Biology of Belief, T. Colin Campbell, author of The China Study, and James Chestnut, developer of the Innate Lifestyle™ and the highly acclaimed Wellness Certification Program, a concept known as "epi-genetics" empowers people to take control of their health by making lifestyle choices that may override their genetic code. Behavior, environment, and our perceptions can affect how our genes are expressed.

Research is proving that if your family has a history of cancer, there are things you can do to bathe the so-called "dis-ease causing" gene in a healthy environment that will suppress the expression of pathology, or altered physiology. This means our genes may produce healthy cells instead of diseased or cancerous cells.

I know, you probably have your mouth wide open and the bottom of your jaw is hitting the floor. Genes do control our chemistry but genes don't control genes. And the chemistry of our body can actually affect or even control our genes. That is why we have to train our body and mind like spiritual warriors. Our training and habits are the food for genes.

Choosing to view life with a positive attitude, eating fruits and vegetables, and moving like an animal, are some of the practices that make up our best offense to expressing our best self! We don't have to be a prisoner of our genes.

FOOD SCIENCE

Food, they say, is an emotional topic, and nowhere is this fact of our modern era more evident than in the constant controversy surrounding types of diets. What we're supposed to eat has become an incredibly confusing question. We have the Paleolithic diet, the Kosher diet, the Rainbow diet, the Zone diet, Weight Watchers, a vegan diet, a vegetarian diet, the South Beach diet, the raw food diet, the Rastafarian diet, the Ornish diet, the Macrobiotic diet, the Mediterranean diet, the low-protein diet, the low-fat diet, the low-carb diet, the non- GMO (genetically modified diet), the junk food diet, the grapefruit diet, the gluten-free diet, the Atkins diet, the Body-type diet, the Blood-type diet, the Ayurvedic diet, the Diet for a New America, the Fruitarian diet, and about a thousand more. I apologize if I left any of your favorites off this list.

The question of "What to eat?" should be common sense. How about eating real food for starters. The hard part in doing this is to get the ego along with its desires, impulses, and needs out of the way. Our fast food mentality, along with the industrialization of food, is creating havoc on not just on our digestive system, but also our entire body-mind constitution.

Eating food that we shouldn't feed our pets has led to a massive rise in heart disease, obesity, diabetes, mental disturbances, decreased immunity and more. Sure, jelly-filled doughnuts look and taste amazing! I know that a hot slice of New York style thin crust cheese pizza might be one of the best inventions in history, maybe more important than the wheel. And I know that ice cream hits the spot right after dinner. But these types of food may lead to an increase in insulin resistant cells, causing diabetes, obesity, and cardiovascular accidents when consumed over a long period of time. Look back at the indigenous Indians of the Americas or the Aborigines of Australia. These people were fit! They were strong! They had great teeth! They had a deep respect for the Earth and the animals that lived on its surface. When they were introduced to the modern refined-style diet, their health changed. They got sick! We have to get back to the days when food was medicine and nourished our body instead of ravaging it.

We should approach food with holistic and vitalistic eyes, because the food we eat becomes the new You. We want to consume foods that encourage moving our cells toward vitality. Many diets exist because people have adopted unhealthy lifestyles and eating habits. The health, rather sick statistics prove it. The top killers in America are considered to be diseases of civilization, or diseases of lifestyle. That means they can be prevented and eradicated by changing our habits. We are shocked when our body begins to show signs and symptoms. Instead of correcting unhealthy eating habits, or eating real whole foods, we take drugs to cover up the expressions (signs or symptoms) of the body that tell us something isn't working correctly. We have within us a $10 million navigation system that speaks to us at any given moment. We need to tune in and listen to the messages.

Think of a dog, for example. When a dog doesn't feel well it eats grass until it throws up. Then the dog drinks from the water bowl, finds some shade, rests and recuperates. We give the dog a belly rub and the dog feels better. Genius idea. Unlike our wise dogs, we traditionally either ignore the messages, or take something to cover up the symptoms. That's because we have been trained to not trust our body's self-healing drive.

"High-tech tomatoes. Mysterious milk. Super-squash. Are we supposed to eat this stuff? Or is it going to eat us?"

Annita Manning

If after eating certain types of we develop rashes by our eyes, our skin is itchy, our bowel movements are painful and few and far between, our joints are achy, or have trouble sleeping, then maybe our body is sensitive to that substance. After eating, listen inward to the human navigation system. Ask yourself, how does my body feel? Am I light or heavy? Am I gassy? Am I straining at the toilet? What's the color of my poop? How does my poop smell? Gross, I know, but extremely valuable information.

If we were Stone Age hunters and gatherers, we would know exactly what to eat. We would know what berries were good at giving us a boost of energy and which ones gave us a psychedelic experience. We would know that certain plants filled us up fully and gave us a timely bowel movement, while others were poisonous and made us vomit. And if we ate woolly mammoth meat, we probably wouldn't be hungry for a couple days. Now is the time to listen to our amazing internal awareness.

So perhaps *The Spinechecker's Manifesto, Vol. II* will be dedicated to food and wellness nutrition, but in the meantime try these suggestions.

View your body as a shrine; as a temple; as a tabernacle.
It's sacred. If you were to make an offering of fruit, incense or flowers to your holy alter it should be of the finest ingredients. You wouldn't offer up a half-eaten rotten apple, stinky incense, or rancid flowers. Your prayer may get rejected! Food should be like an offering to your body.

FOOD SCIENCE *(cont.)*

Go organic.
That means no pesticides, herbicides, fungicides, insecticides, or anything else that ends in an "-ides." Anything that ends in an "-ides" means it is designed to kill something...including us.

Eat mostly plants, fruits and vegetables.
The more colorful the better! They contain most of the vitamins and minerals your body needs.

If you choose to eat other animals... make sure you can kill it yourself.
With this suggestion you will have to look deep within your hunter and gatherer being and ask yourself if you have what it takes to kill a fish... a chicken... a buffalo... an ostrich... daisy the cow... a lamb. If you can kill it, then you can eat it.

"It would be nice if the Food and Drug Administration stopped issuing warnings about toxic substances and just gave me the names of one or two things still safe to eat."

Robert Fuoss

Choose wild-free range.
That means the animal isn't kept in overcrowded conditions and is free to eat and roam off the land. If you are going to eat meat, say a chicken for example, do you want to eat a chicken that is so cramped in her quarters, that her legs are mangled and deformed, she sits in poop, and can't open her wings? Or would you rather eat a chicken that has a chance to roam around the farm and play "chicken" with Daisy the cow? Your call.

Stay off of refined sugar.
I know...it is hard, but it creates destruction, not only of your teeth, but also of the body.

Get 15 minutes a day of sunlight.
Get your sun energy! The body produces Vitamin D from sunlight and excessive seclusion from the sun can lead to deficiency. A lack of sunlight is considered to be one of the primary causes of seasonal affective disorder (SAD), a serious form of the "winter blues". So bask in the sun and prevent turning blue.

Eat whole grains.
That includes quinoa, barley, millet, and oats. Some people have sensitively to wheat as a result of gluten sensitivity, so maybe you want to reduce wheat consumption. If it has refined in the title, maybe you pass on it.

You can definitely make an argument for supplementing with omega-3's.
Study after study has shown the necessity of having a diet rich in Omega-3s for proper neurological and cardiovascular function. Fish oils aren't the only oils rich in Omega-3s. Flax, hemp, purslane, evening primrose, walnut, pumpkin, borage and more are rich in Omega-3, and are options if someone can't kill their own fish.

You can definitely make an argument for supplementing with spirulina, & chlorella.
Chlorella and spirulina are some of the most amazing food sources on planet Earth. Spirulina is a tiny aquatic plant that has been eaten by humans since prehistoric times. It contains 60 - 70% all-vegetable protein, essential vitamins and phytonutrients such as the antioxidant beta-carotene, the rare essential fatty acid Gamma-linoleic acid (GLA), and

more goodies. Spirulina is rich in iron, magnesium and trace minerals, and has easier-to-absorb forms of iron than iron supplements. It also contains very high levels of calcium. In addition, Spirulina is one of the few plant sources of Vitamin B12. That's great news for vegetarians who don't get Vitamin B12 because of not eating meat! Chlorella is the richest source of chlorophyll yet known, which is useful in ridding the body of toxins, including heavy metals (like mercury in dental fillings), and cleansing the bowel, liver and bloodstream. All green leafy vegetables contain chlorophyll, but none contain as much as Chlorella, gram for gram.

Limit the amount of packaged foods.
Eating fresh real food, versus processed packaged foods may allow your body to function at a higher level. I like real ingredients versus artificial ingredients.

Stay off of soft drinks.
Several scientific studies have provided experimental evidence that soft drinks are bad for your teeth and bones and leads to acidosis.. That's just the half of it!

Drink plentiful amounts water.
Our body is composed of 70% water. Our brain is composed of water. Our vertebral discs are composed of water. Our muscles are composed of water. You get the point. Our bodies are composed of water, so it is essential to stay hydrated so you can stay afloat.

"Do vegetarians eat animal crackers?"

Author Unknown

Follow the 93/7 % or 86/14 %rule.
This is a modification of the 80/20% rule, which says, 'eat well 80% of the time, and 20% you can enjoy the pleasures of your palette and enjoy the things you know you should not be eating regularly.' This removes the guilt from eating your pizza, your doughnut, or your cookie. So if you eat well 6 days out of the week and one day you eat off the path, that means 86 % of the time you are eating well, and 14% off the path. If you eat well for 13 days and one day you take off to drink some beers and have a pizza, that would be 93 % of the time you are on the mark and 7 % off. Sometimes you are a B+. Sometimes you are an A-. If you want to be an A+ then you know what you have to do to excel at that level.

Eating food should not create more dis-stress in your life.
Changing habits is hard. Overcoming the old impulses and desires is hard. That is where will power and discipline comes in. This new attitude of healthy eating or wellness nutrition will crease positive stress, called eu-stress. In time your new eating habits will create a stronger and more powerful YOU.

GUIDE TO DEEP & RESTFUL SLEEP

Bedtime Preparation Flow

Don't Change Your Sleep Time

Connect to the rhythm of life by going to bed at the same time every day. We have an innately intelligent system that loves repetition and routine. If we make it a habit to go to sleep at the same time every night, we create a groove or impression in our brain. The deeper the groove the easier it is to access it.

Get to Bed as Early as Possible

By going to bed early we give our body time to recuperate. Melatonin secretion from the pineal gland starts around 9:00 pm and ends around 7:30 am (Melatonin facilitates our sleep). Also, our organs, muscles, and glands do a majority of their growth and repair during the night. If we interrupt our sleep, detoxification and purification can't occur efficiently. The result is a groggy, sluggish body. Get to bed as early as possible to stay recharged and energized.

Create a Nest

Go primal. Make your bedroom like a cave, just like our hunter and gatherer ancestors did. Your bed should be comfortable, nurturing and safe. It should be a place where you can feel protected from all types of predators.

Sleep in Complete Darkness

When light hits the eyes, it activates the pineal gland and disrupts the production of melatonin. Remember melatonin secretion from the pineal gland starts around 9:00 pm and ends around 7:30 am. That means you should be getting very very sleepy during this period of time. Close your blinds to block out any streetlights or any electrical devices near the bed.

Keep Your Bed for Sleeping

This takes us back to the idea of creating a sleeping ritual. Once we slide under the sheets the body innately knows it is time for shuteye, and begins to tune out to the conscious world. Watching television or working in bed is counterproductive to the sleeping process.

Remove the Residue of the Day and Take a Warm Bath or Shower Before Bed

Taking a shower or bath is not only relaxing, but it washes off the dirt of the day. Go to bed fresh.

Start a Nightly Contemplative Practice

Ask your 'Self' how you behaved today. Were you positive and constructive in the way you communicated with your self and others, or were you destructive in your thoughts, emotions, and actions? Checking in allows you to make a mental adjustment for the next day. This is a deep and powerful spiritual practice to make repair and regeneration to any one you may have harmed or who has harmed you. This may help you go to bed with a clear mind.

GUIDE TO DEEP & RESTFUL SLEEP *(cont.)*

Listen to Delta Wave Sleeping Music
As we sleep we will pass through several states where the brain is functioning at a certain frequency. Delta wave is the most relaxing and deepest state of sleep. Listening to delta wave sleeping music prepares you to enter deep sleep. For more information go to www.neuroacoustic.com and learn about the outstanding work of Dr. Jeffrey Thompson.

Wear Socks to Bed
Keep your feet warm through the night by wearing socks since your feet tend to get the coldest the fastest of any body part as a result of poorer circulation. Since our body temperature is at its warmest around 7:00 pm and is at the lowest by 4:30 am, keep your temperature consistent. Bedtime is the time when you actually want your feet to fall asleep!

Practice Daily Breathing Sequences
Keep your stress levels down throughout the day by focusing on your breath. Follow the sequences in this manifesto to keep your breath flowing and your mind calm.

No TV Right before Bed
TV can be stimulating. Sleep preparation should be calming. So maybe turn off the tube a few hours before sleep. And definitely don't watch the news right before you go to bed unless you want to fill your brain with the worst images and occurrences around the world. That could be stressful and prevent you from falling asleep.

Read Something Spiritual or Relaxing
This goes along with the theme of keeping calm, relaxed, and breathing deeply. Reading the new Harry Potter book or a Dan Brown (Da Vinci's Code), may keep you up for hours.

Just do it. Orgasms Increase Endorphins
Endorphins help you reach deep sleep. Now you have a scientific reason to have sex.

Don't Eat a Late Dinner.
Keep in mind that the body suspends bowel movements around 10:30pm. Eating an early dinner ensures a bowel movement before bedtime. According to our innate circadian rhythm, a bowel movement is most likely to occur around 8:30pm. In order to ensure we don't have an undigested meal sitting in our belly while we sleep, try to eat early.

"People who say they sleep like a baby usually don't have one."

Leo J. Burke

Wake Up Flow

Avoid Using Loud Alarm Clocks
A loud alarm causes you to activate your flight or flight/ sympathetic nervous system. This isn't the ideal way to wake up. Try the Zen Alarm Clock which wakes you up with a

chime. Or, if you have an iPhone you can download an application for a chime alarm that does the same thing. Another fantastic option is a sun clock alarm, which simulates the sun rising by getting brighter as you get close to your wake up time.

Take a Couple Deep Breaths

Just lie in bed for a few moments and take some deep breaths. This should get you into the present moment and into your body.

Do Yoga

Clear out a space in your home where you can begin to move and breathe in rhythm. Get your energy flowing as you become acutely aware of how your body mind feels as you begin the day. You may realize that you are exploding with energy or you may find that you need to take it easy. The morning is a great time to take inventory of how you move and feel.

"A good laugh and a long sleep are the best cures in the doctor's book."

Irish Proverb

During the Day Flow

Get Daily Exercise

Exercise helps your body run more efficiently. If your physiological processes are running properly, your sleep should also be more efficient. Try not to exercise too close to your bedtime as that may keep you charged up.

Listen to Relaxation CDs

Dr. Jeffrey Thompson has created a line of CDs to enter into a relaxed state during the day. Try his Ultimate Nap CD for your mid day siesta! It has a 10, 20, and 30-minute option!

Avoid Caffeine

If you have trouble sleeping, avoid caffeine. You may be a person who is not able to effectively breakdown caffeine, which means it stays in your system for a long time. Even a mid day cup of java may keep you up at night. Definitely stay away from caffeine at night unless you are in Spain and trying to keep up with the Spaniards way of life.

Avoid Alcohol

Even though alcohol can make you sleepy, it interferes with the body's ability to reach deep sleep. Getting into a sustained state of deep sleep is necessary for health. Just like caffeine, avoid drinking alcohol too late at night, unless you are in Italy on vacation.

Do Breathing, Concentration, and Meditation Sequences

Connect to a higher vibrational source by drawing your attention inward. When you withdraw your senses from the outer world and place your attention on your breath, stress levels are diminished. By decreasing the accumulation of stress throughout the day you'll experience less stress at night before you go to sleep.

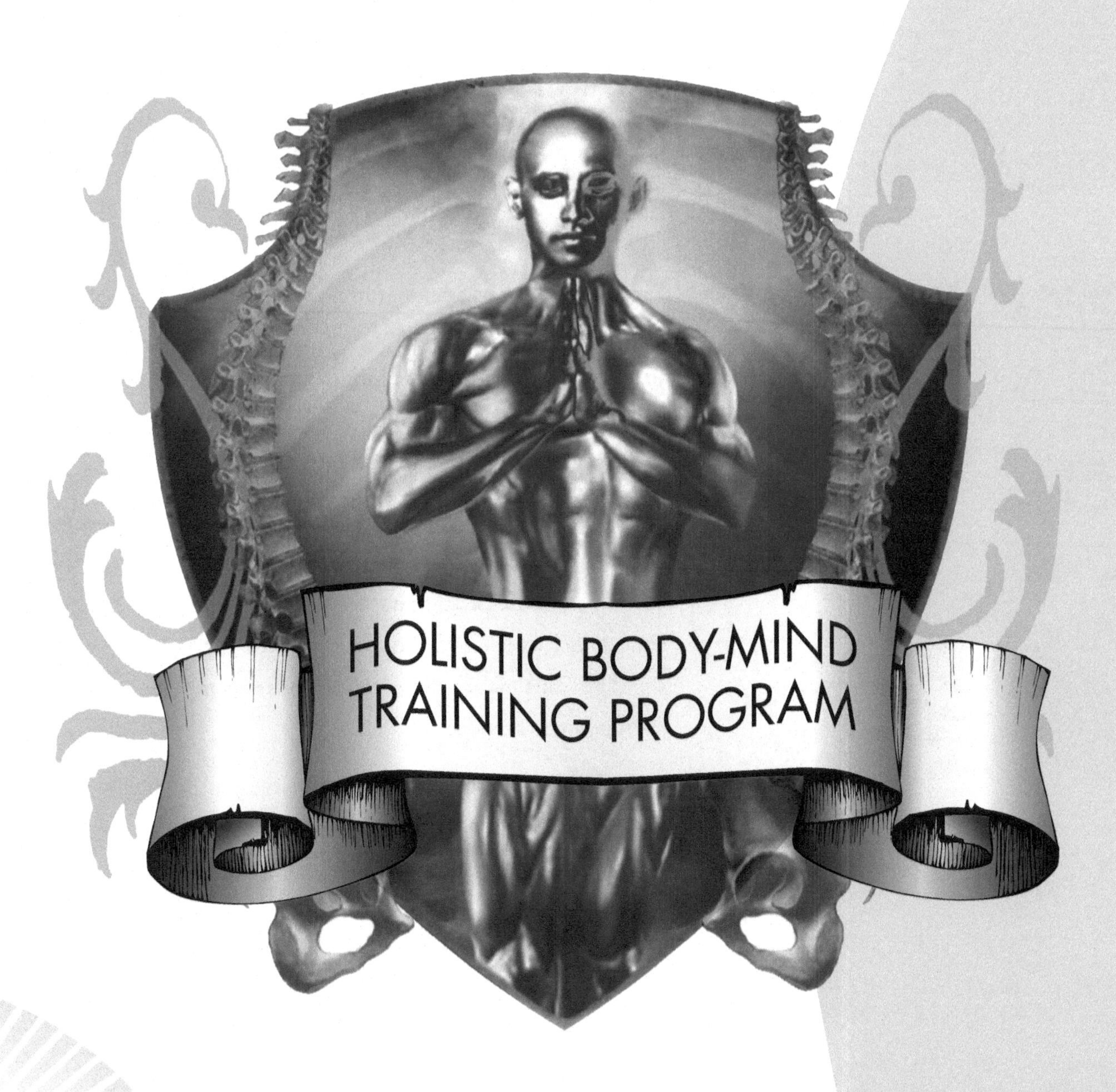
HOLISTIC BODY-MIND
TRAINING PROGRAM

GENERAL INSTRUCTIONS

To receive the maximum benefit from the sequences in this manifesto, practice with consistency. A great time to practice is first thing in the morning when you have an empty stomach, colon and bladder. If you practice them in the afternoon, make sure you have adequate time to digest any food you have eaten. Wait about two hours after eating a light meal and up to four after a heavy meal. Feel free to repeat the sequences as often as possible throughout the day, especially if you sit in a chair for extended periods or live an active lifestyle.

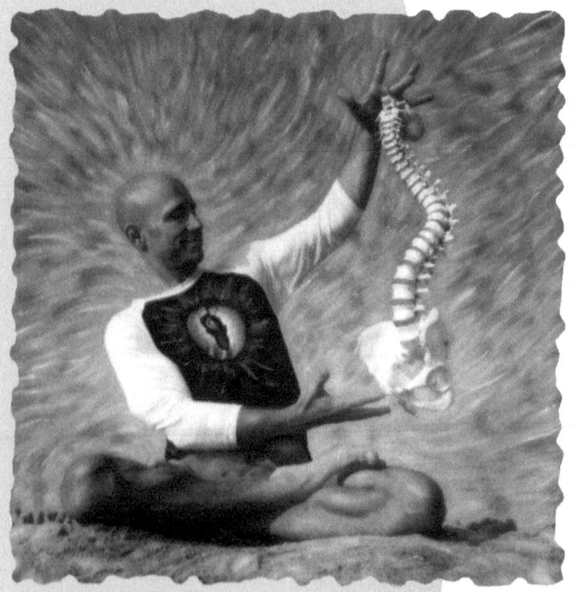

The sequences are not demanding athletically, although some may prove to be confronting and challenging based on your past traumas, physical and emotional limitations, and current lifestyle. These sequences should improve your posture, increase your flexibility, and promote the relaxation response.

Although your body-mind will receive benefit from consistent practice of these sequences, please collaborate and consult with your health care-practitioner to ensure that they are congruent with your unique constitution, and not contraindicated for your present situation. This manifesto is not designed to replace professional instruction or advice.

With the **movement sequences** you can do multiple repetitions. Try 5-10 in each direction. You can also "hold" the movement for 1-5 breaths, or you can let movement flow with the breath. Optimally you will be doing these movements throughout the day.

With the **stretching sequences**, try doing 3-5 sets. You can hold each position for a short stretch or a long stretch. A short stretch would be about 5-8 breaths and a long stretch would be about 25 breaths.

With the core **strengthening sequences**, try doing 3-5 sets of 25 repetitions.

THE ROAD TO WELLNESS

Phase 1
(0 - 6 weeks)

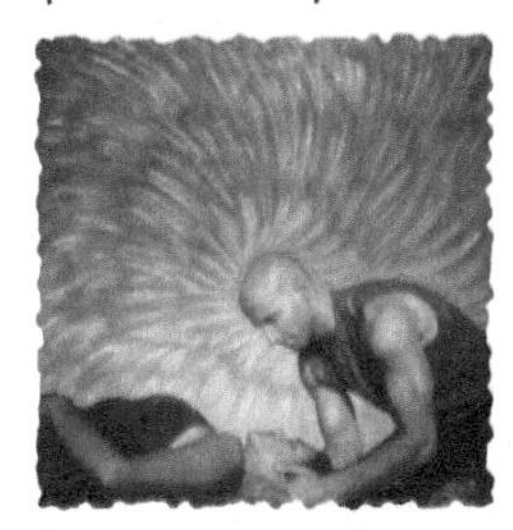

Repair	Repetition
Specific Scientific Chiropractic Adjustments	*3 - 5 times per week*
Basic Full Spine Movement Sequences	*3 - 5 times per day*
Basic Full Spine Stretching Sequences	*3 - 5 times per day*
Spinal Pump/Cannonballs	*every hour of the day*
Cervical Traction/Yoga Backbender (week 3 – 4)	*3 - 5 times per week*
Breathing, Concentration, Meditation, Affirmations	*1- 3 times per day*

Phase 2
(6 - 24 weeks, and up to 12 months)

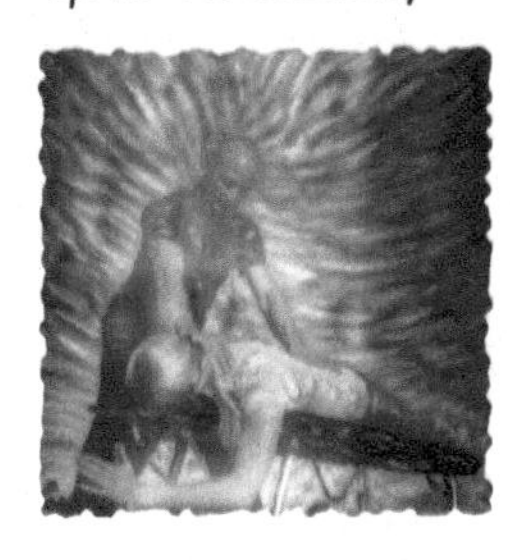

Remodeling	Repetition
Specific Scientific Chiropractic Adjustments	*2 - 3 times per week*
Basic Full Spine Movement Sequences	*3 - 5 times per day*
Basic Full Spine Stretching Sequences	*3 - 5 times per day*
Core Strengthening Sequences	*3 - 5 times per day*
Spinal Pump/Cannonballs	*every hour of the day*
Cervical Traction/Yoga Backbender	*3 - 5 times per week*
Breathing, Concentration, Meditation, Affirmations	*1 -3 times per day*

Phase 3
(For the rest of your life)

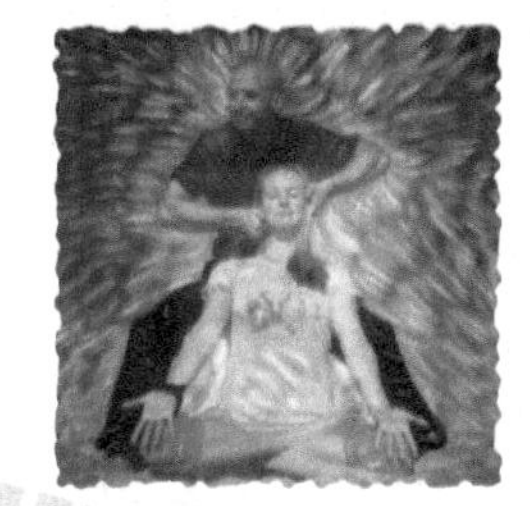

Optimizing	Repetition
Specific Scientific Chiropractic Adjustments	*Determined by Lifestyle*
Basic Full Spine Movement Sequences	*3 - 5 times per day*
Basic Full Spine Stretching Sequences	*3 - 5 times per day*
Basic Full Spine Strengthening Sequences	*3 - 5 times per day*
Spinal Pump/Cannonballs	*every hour of the day*
Cervical Traction/Yoga Backbender	*3 - 5 times per week*
Breathing, Concentration, Meditation, Affirmations	*1- 3 times per day*

TYPES OF CARE

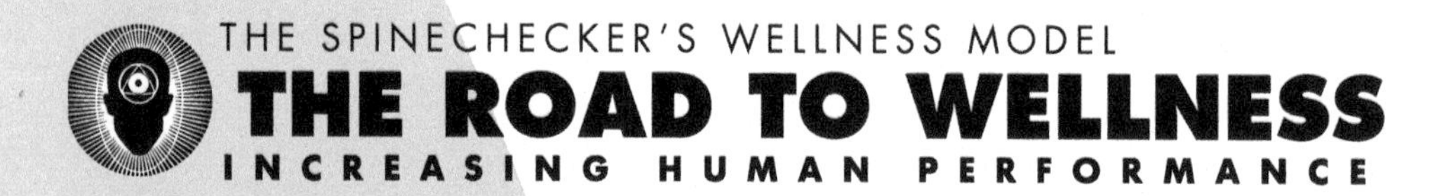

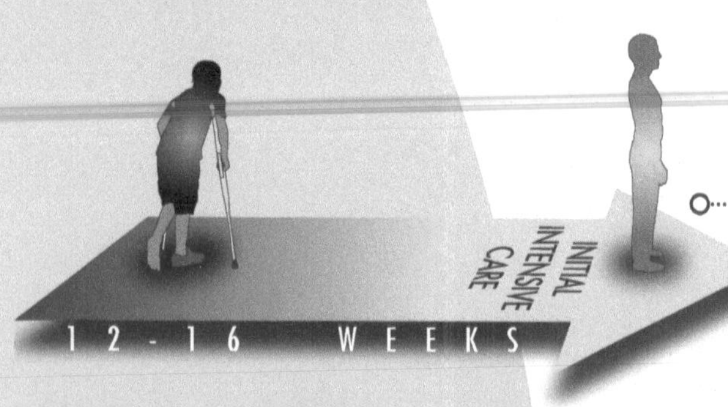

INITIAL INTENSIVE CARE

This stage of care is designed to stabilize your spine and to begin to improve its function as quickly as possible.

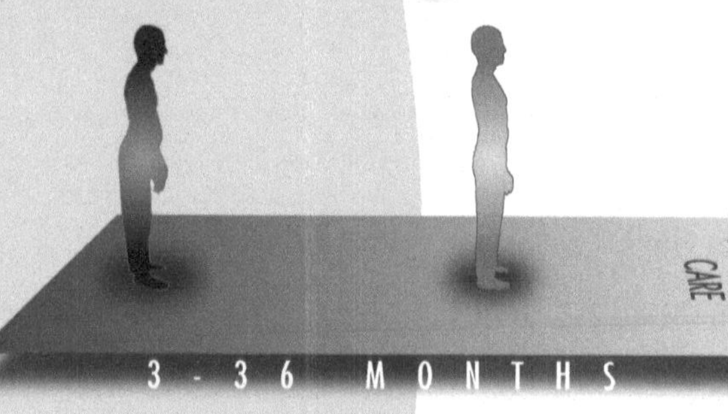

CORRECTIVE CARE

This is the phase to retrain your abnormal movement patterns and return your spine as near as possible to 'normal' function.

MAINTENANCE CARE

Maintenance care involves ongoing **SPINECHECKS** to maintain the function of your spine, correcting Vertebral Subluxations as you create them.

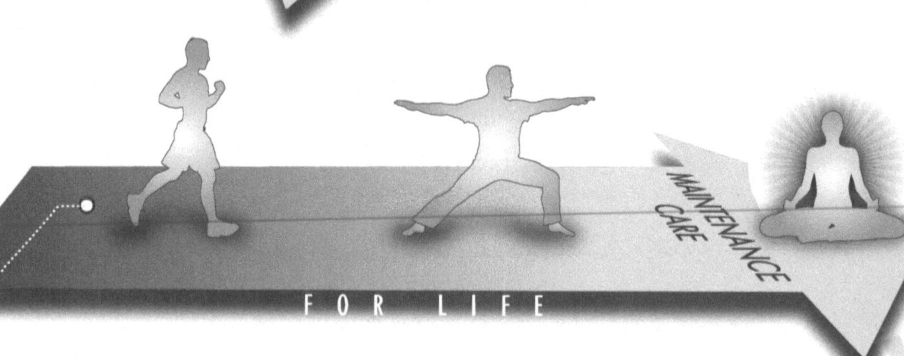

THE SPINECHECKER'S WELLNESS MODEL

HOLISTIC BODY-MIND TRAINING PROGRAM

WORDS OF WISDOM

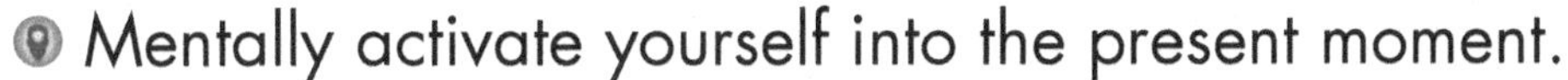

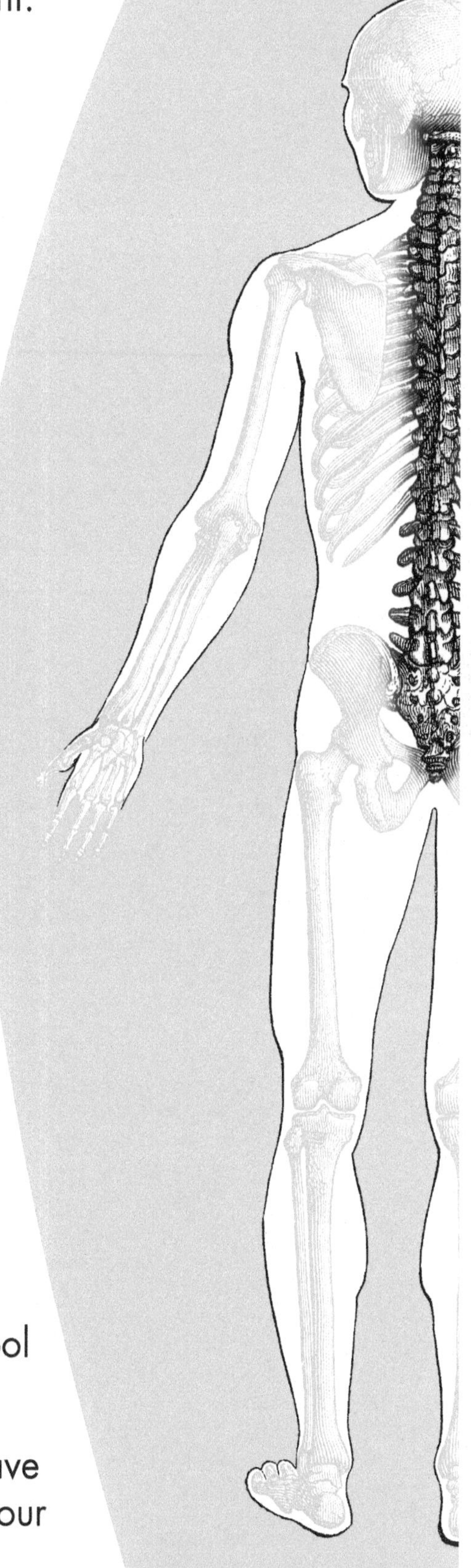

- Mentally activate yourself into the present moment.
- Relax as deeply as you can.
- Breathe freely and consciously.
- Link all fluid movements with your breath.
- Move your body with respect.
- Move incrementally...slowly.
- If it hurts, back off.
- If you feel restriction... don't force it.
- If you feel pain, dizziness, or nausea... stop... and consult your chiropractor immediately.
- After completing each sequence of movements...relax...breathe...and expand!
- Remember, it is your birthright to have a powerful spine!
- Your breathing/moving sequences should be fluid and enjoyable, steady and comfortable. There is no struggle in true yogic asana.
- The barometer of your breathing/moving sequences is the quality of your breath.
- Allow the breathing/moving sequences to be a tool for observing of how you care for your body.
- If your breathing has been disturbed, or you have become agitated, take a small rest and refocus your attention on your breath.

ENERGETIC FLOW CHART

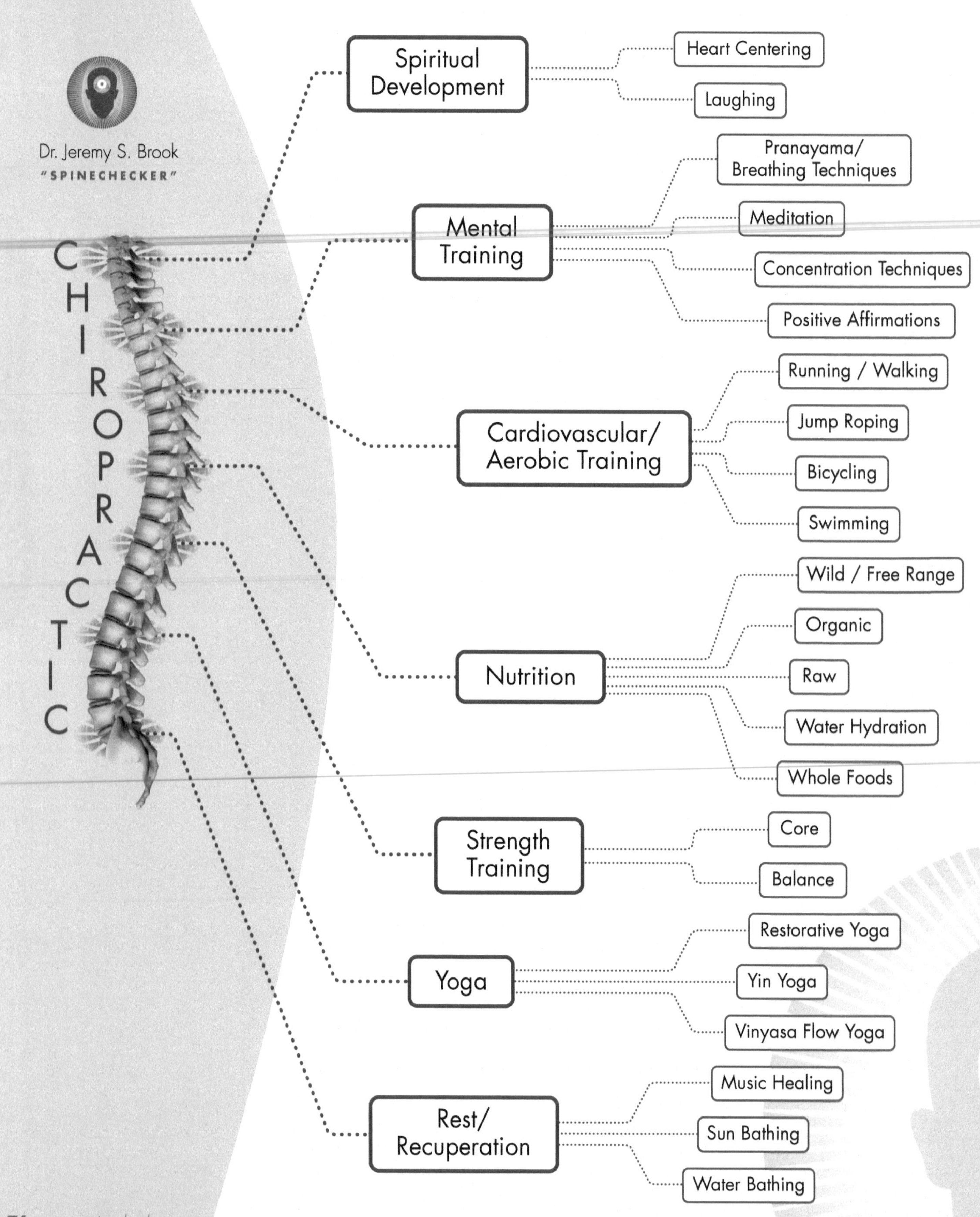

THE SPINECHECKER'S WELLNESS MODEL

ILLNESS/WELLNESS CONTINUUM

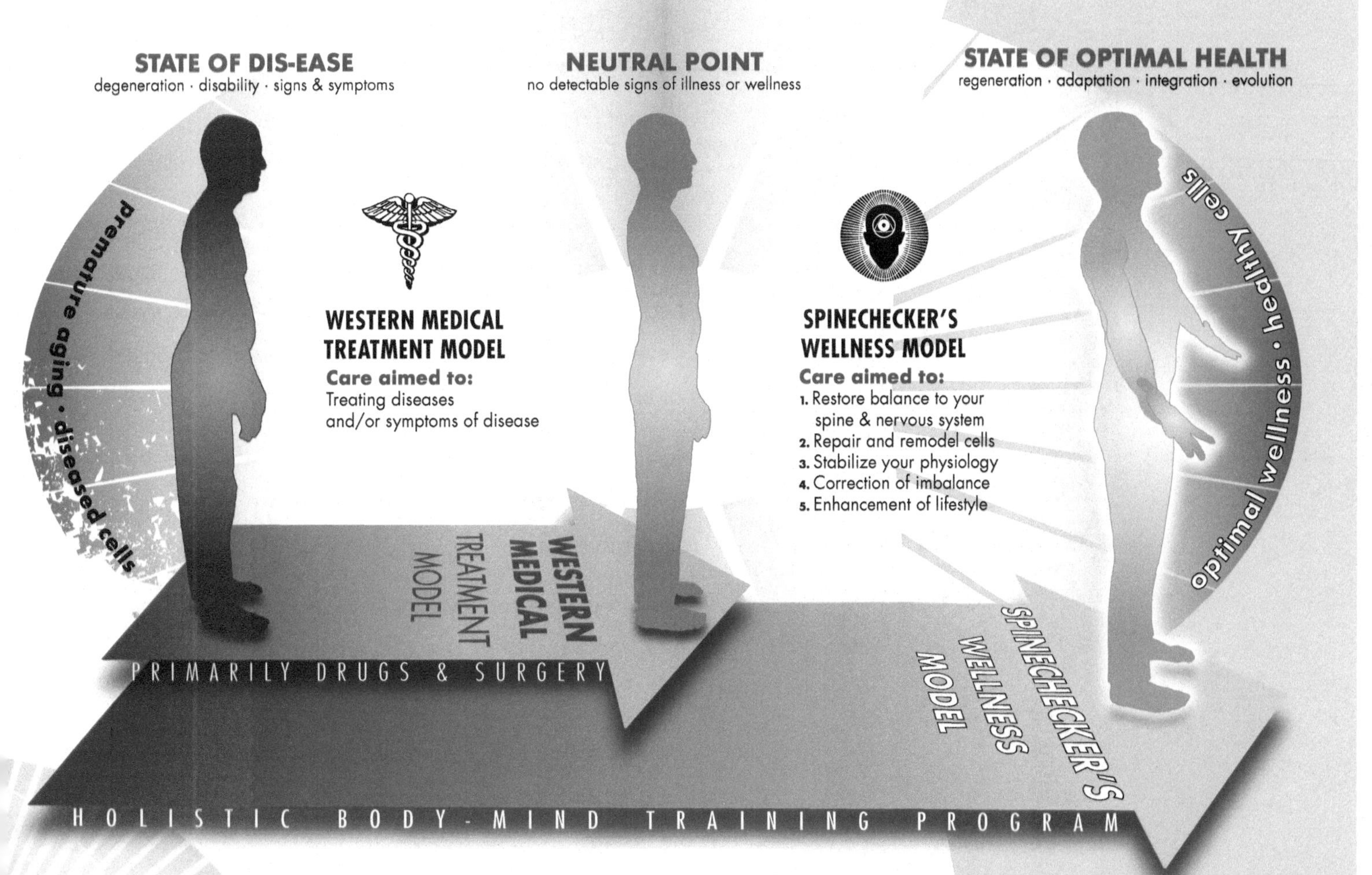

BASIC POINTERS FOR A STRONG TADASANA {MOUNTAIN POSE}

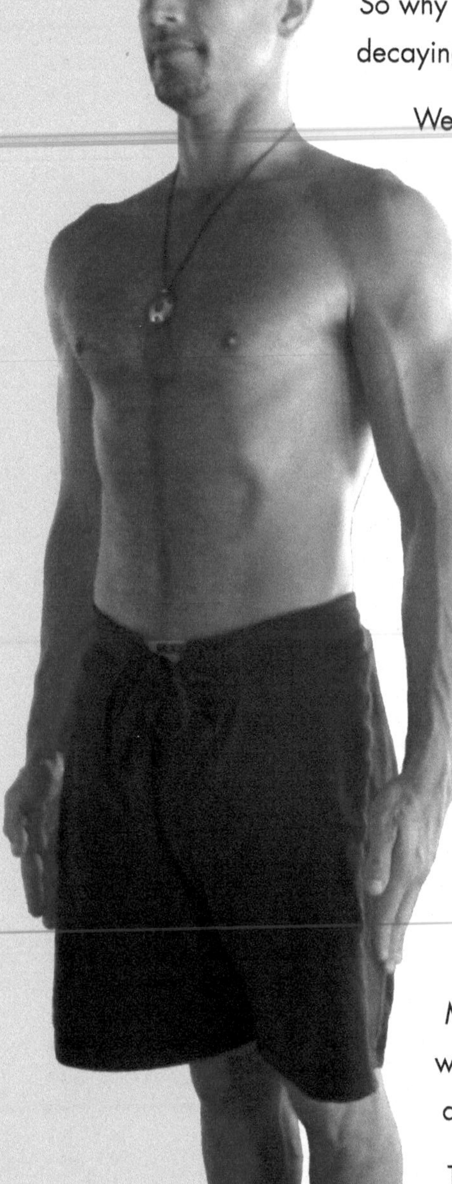

The great modern yoga master, B.K.S. Iyengar, once said "You want to stand on your head and you don't even know how to stand on your feet."

So why should we care how we stand tall? Because the body is always decaying!

We live for roughly nine months in a water filled universe.... only to squeeze out of a small opening...if we're lucky.... and then we are subjected to the stressful and powerful effects of gravity. As we get older, we then live a life crammed into a chair for 16 hours a day. On top of that we have to follow a set of moral and ethical codes. It's hard work to be alive.

And that is why we have to stand tall! With our feet rooted into the Earth, our pelvis level, our heart open, and our head on our shoulders with all eyes open we learn to develop strength, courage, vitality, awareness, and total oneness with the universe.

To demonstrate how to stand correctly, we'll use the yogic model of standing tall ... the classic pose Tadasana, or Mountain Pose.

Tadasana is a seemingly simple pose. It seems so basic and obvious, that most of us don't give it the time and attention it deserves.

My recommendation is to remember to remember! When you are waiting at a crosswalk, assume Tadasana. When you are in line at Whole Foods...become Mountain Pose.

The more you practice this pose, the more you will align your "self" against the stresses of gravity. With correct alignment your body will be more energy efficient and strain free. The less stress...the less tension...the less dis-ease...the less degeneration... the more ease...the more energy...the more regeneration!

"Start by stopping."

Chuck Miller

BASIC POINTERS FOR A STRONG TADASANA {MOUNTAIN POSE} *(cont.)*

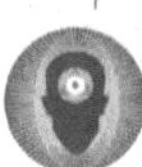

BREATHE!

Inhale from the lowest part of your spine up through the top of your head.

Focus on all the points mentioned above as you breathe.

Feel the effects of correct alignment.

HEAD

Move your skull backward so that the middle of your ear lines up with the middle of your shoulders.

Focus your eye gaze on one point straight ahead.

HEART CENTER

Lift your inner sternum up.

Feel the expansion in the area between the back of your sternum and the front of your spine.

Broaden across your collarbones.

SHOULDER BLADES

Relax your shoulders away from your ears.

Feel your shoulder blades move down your back.

ARMS

Straighten your elbows and point your fingers down toward the floor.

NAVEL CENTER

Locate a point roughly 2 inches below your belly button and draw it inward by gently contracting your abdominal muscles.

LOWER RIBS

Draw your lower ribs inward by contracting your upper abdominals.

TAILBONE

Release your tailbone and sacrum down toward the floor by contracting your pelvic floor muscles.

KNEES

Unlock your knees by bending them slightly.

Draw your kneecaps up by contracting your quadriceps.

Find the middle point between the knee-bend and the locked-knee.

Relax your buttocks.

FEET

Lift and spread your toes wide.

Observe the arch created in your foot.

Lower your toes down while maintaining the arch.

BASIC MOVEMENTS OF THE CERVICAL SPINE

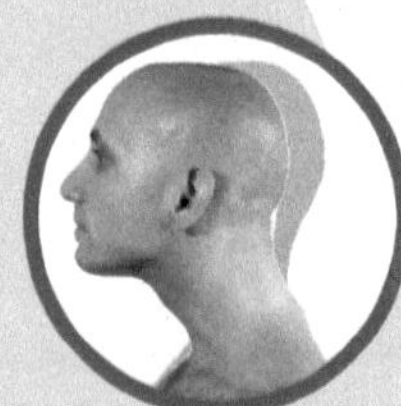

FUNKY CHICKEN • Extension of the Skull

Intention - To lubricate the joint between your skull and top vertebrae (Atlanto-Occipital Joint)

Movement -

Keeping your chin parallel to the floor, gently glide your chin forward.

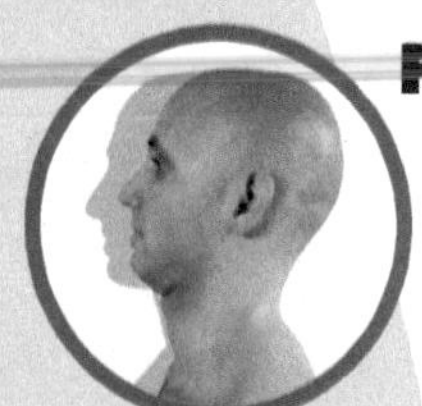

FUNKY CHICKEN • Flexion of the Skull

Intention - To lubricate the joint between your skull and top vertebrae (Atlanto-Occipital Joint).

Movement -

Keeping your chin parallel to the floor, gently glide your chin backward.

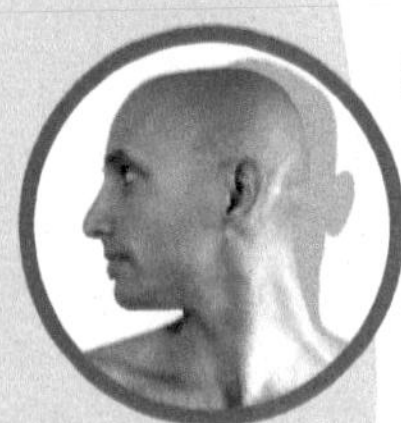

SIDE TO SIDE • Rotation

Intention - To lubricate, primarily, the joints between the top 2 vertebrae in the spine, the atlas and axis, as well as the rest of the cervical spine.

Movement -

On the exhale, while keeping your chin parallel to the floor, look over your right shoulder.
Return your head to center on the inhale and repeat to the left side.

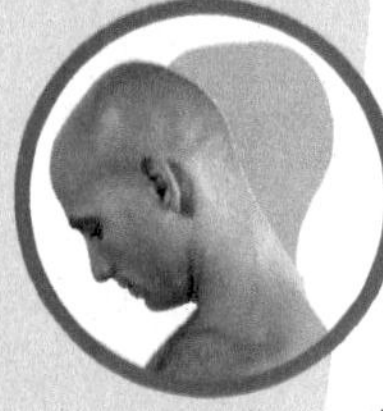

CHIN TO CHEST • Flexion

Intention - Lubrication of all the joints of the neck.

Movement -

On the exhale, gently bow your forehead to your chest.

KEYPOINT: Remember to keep your sternum lifted.

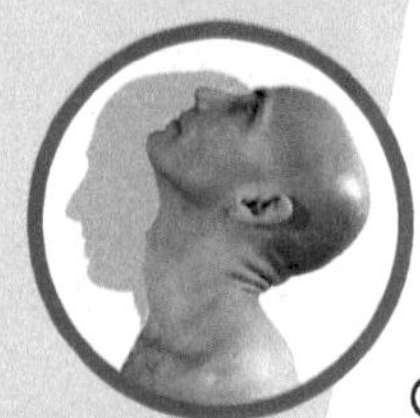

CHIN TO SKY • Extension

Intention - Lubrication of all the joints of the neck.

Movement -

On the inhale, gently raise your chin to the sky.

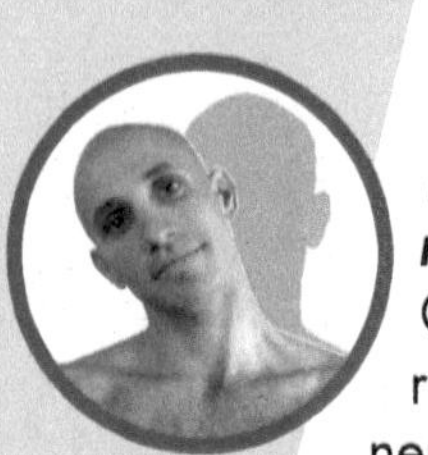

EAR TO SHOULDER • Lateral Flexion

Intention - Lubrication of all the joints of the neck.

Movement -

On the exhale, gently release your right ear to your right shoulder. On the inhale return your head to a neutral position.

KEYPOINT: Keep your shoulders relaxed and don't force the movement.

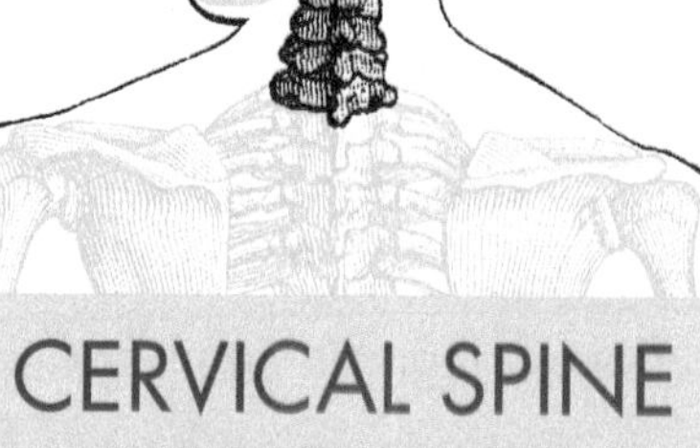

CERVICAL SPINE LUBRICATION

Benefits:

- Increased Flexibility
- Decreased Pain
- Increased Energy
- Increased Creativity and Clarity
- Improved Posture

"Start by Stopping"

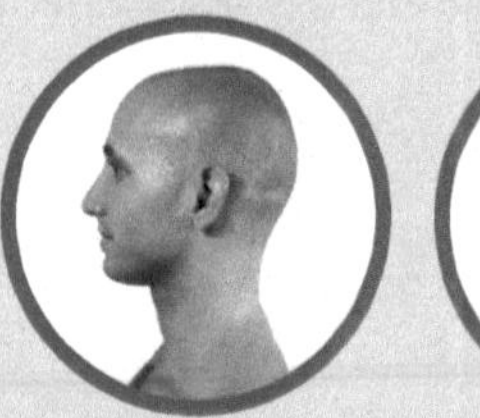

Lateral View *Anterior View*

Views of a Neutral Cervical Spine

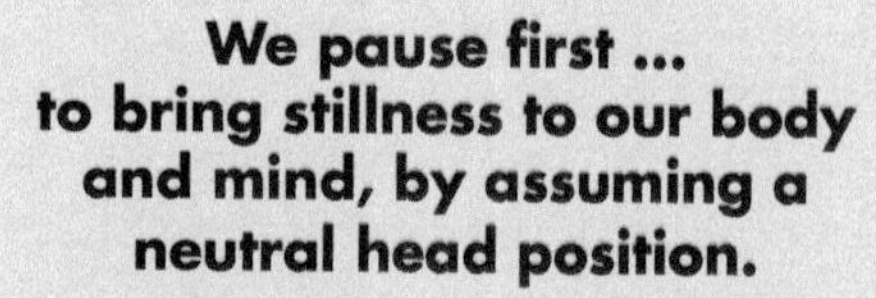

We pause first ... to bring stillness to our body and mind, by assuming a neutral head position.

First, inhale through your nose, and expand your inner sternum out and up.

Next, check the position of your head. Level your eyes so that they are gazing straight ahead.

Gently glide your head backward so that if you were to draw a line down the center of your ear it would bisect the middle of your shoulder.

Relax, expand into your body, and feel the effects.

Now we can begin with the motions of the neck.

ADVANCED MOVEMENTS OF THE UPPER CERVICAL SPINE

FUNKY CHICKEN PLUS FLEXION

Intention - Lubrication of the joints at the top of the neck.

Movement:

1. Retract your chin backward.

2. Lower your chin toward your chest.

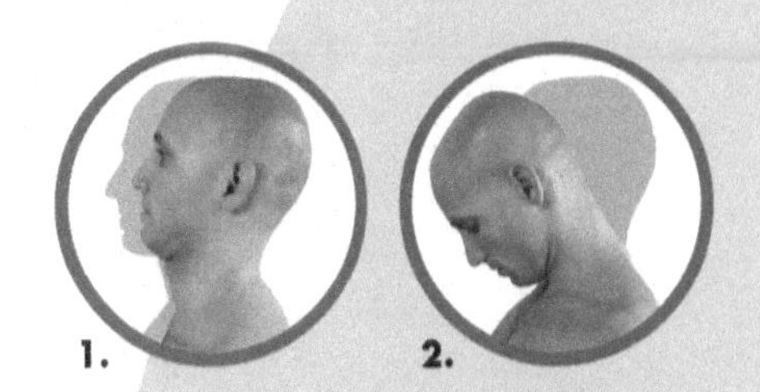

FUNKY CHICKEN PLUS FLEXION PLUS ROTATION

Intention - Lubrication of the joints at the top of the neck.

Movement:

1. Retract your chin backward.

2. Lower your chin toward your chest.

3a & 3b. Slowly rotate your chin to the left.

Return to the center and repeat to the right.

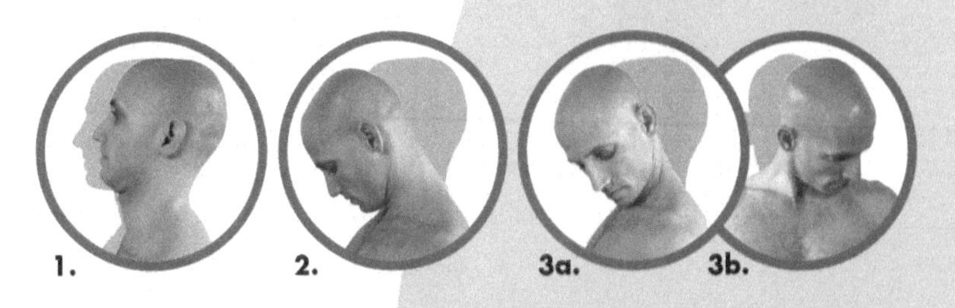

ADVANCED MOVEMENTS OF THE LOWER CERVICAL SPINE

FUNKY CHICKEN PLUS EXTENSION

Intention - Lubrication of the joints at the base of the neck and the top of the shoulders.

Movement:

1. Extend your chin forward.

2. Raise your chin to the sky.

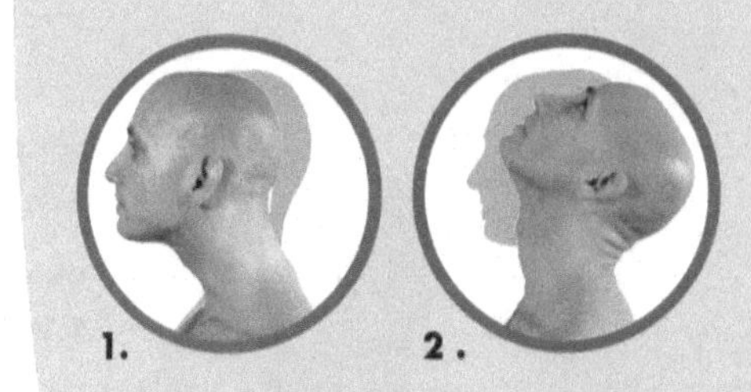

FUNKY CHICKEN PLUS EXTENSION PLUS ROTATION

Intention - Lubrication of the joints at the base of the neck and the top of the shoulders.

Movement:

1. Extend your chin forward.

2. Raise your chin to the sky.

3a & 3b. Slowly rotate your chin to the left

Return to the center and repeat to the right.

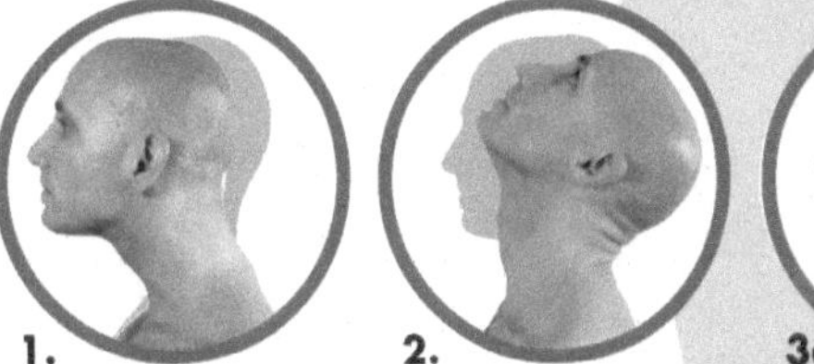

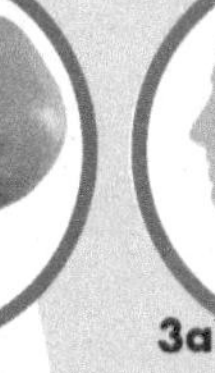

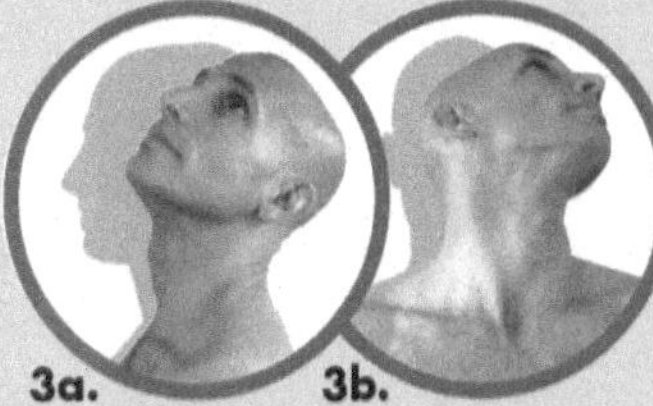

1. 2. 3a. 3b.

CAUTION: ***If you experience dizziness in this position, return your head to a straight forward position and sit down.***

EAR TO SHOULDER PLUS ROTATION

Intention - Lubrication of the joints in the neck.

Movement:

1. On the exhale, gently release your right ear to your right shoulder, halfway.

2. Slowly rotate your chin toward the right shoulder

3. Return your head back to the halfway point and then return your head to center. Repeat on the other side.

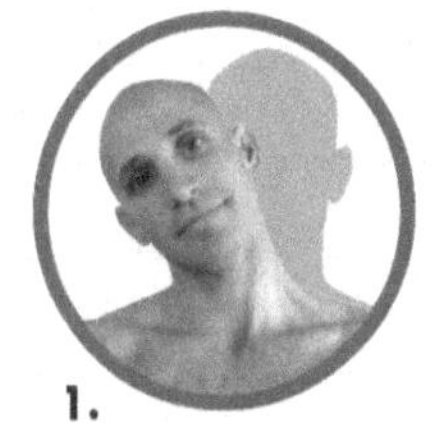

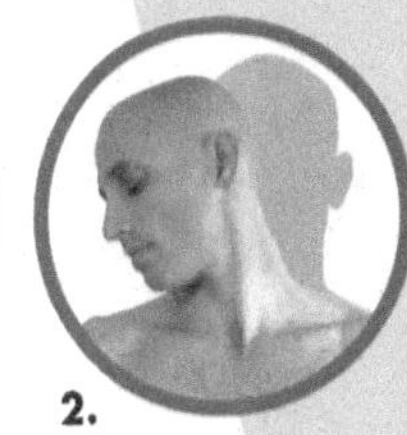

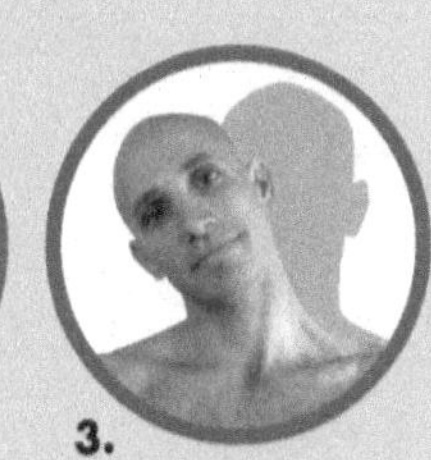

1. 2. 3.

BASIC MOVEMENTS OF THE THORACIC SPINE

CAT TILT • Flexion of the Spine Posterior Rotation of the Pelvis

Intention - To lubricate the joints of the spine, the sacroiliac and hip. To nourish the discs through imbibition (the process of bringing nutrients into the discs through specific movements).

Set Up:
Come onto your hands and knees with your hands underneath your shoulders, or slightly in front of your shoulders. Position your knees under your hip bones.

Movement:
As you exhale, round your spine. Draw your navel in toward your spine, tuck your tailbone under. Point your sit bones toward the floor. Softly lower your chin to your chest.

DOG TILT • Extension of the Spine Anterior Rotation of the Pelvis

Intention - To lubricate the joints of the spine, the sacroiliac and hip. To nourish the discs through imbibition (the process of bringing nutrients into the discs through specific movements).

Set Up:
Begin in the same position as Cat Tilt.

Movement:
As you inhale, arch your spine. Release your spine down toward your navel, lift your tailbone up and point your sit bones upwards. Scoop your inner sternum up toward the sky.

CHILD'S POSE • Flexion

Intention - To lubricate the joints of the spine, sacroiliac, and hips while in a rounded position. To gently traction the spine.

Set Up:
Begin kneeling.

Movement:
On the exhale, fold forward so that your chest lands softly on your thighs.

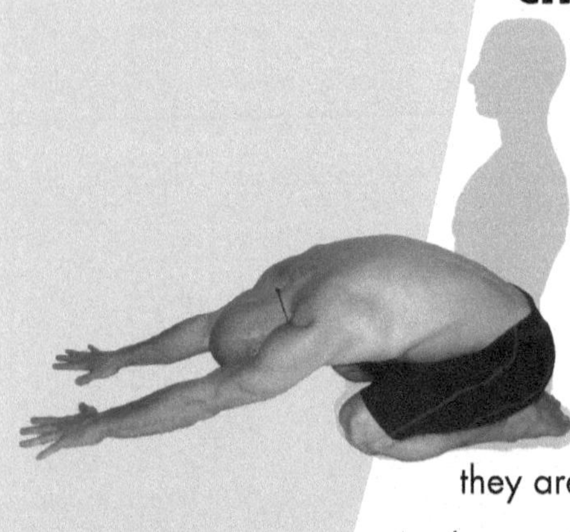

Extend your arms straight out in front of you. Look at your hands to make sure they are in line with your shoulders.

Anchor your hands into the floor by pressing the palms into the floor. Press into your hands to push your sit bones back onto your heels.

THORACIC SPINE LUBRICATION

"Feel Your Heart Beat"

Once you have activated your neck, or your cervical spine, the next step is to **expand the area** in the front and back of your heart.

This region of your spine houses the organs and glands responsible for breathing, digestion, detoxification, and immune support, as well as the muscles that keep your spine erect. Therefore, it is **essential for the restoration and preservation** of one's health that this area be malleable and strong.

So when performing the movements of the mid-back, or your thoracic spine, **remember to first pause**.

Feel your heart center and, from the inside, lift your sternum up and outwards toward the sky. **Energetically, broaden wide** across your collarbones by feeling your chest widen.

Then release your shoulder blades down your back. Find the proper ear to shoulder alignment...and now you are **ready to explore**.

But first... remember to link each movement with your breath. With **intense concentration** you will **activate the intelligence** within your body, and achieve more advanced states of interconnectedness.

So remember to pause ... relax deeply... breathe... and feel the effects.

COBRA & SPHINX • Extension of the Spine

Intention - To lubricate the joints of the mid and low back. To open the heart center and decompress the low back.

Set Up:

1. Lie on your stomach. Begin with your elbows under your shoulders.
2. Gradually extend your hands out in front of you.
(See Variations **1** *-* **3***)*

Movement:

3. On the inhale, press your hands or forearms gently into the floor, arch your spine, and scoop your inner sternum toward the sky.

1.

KEYPOINT: Keep your head relaxed and look straight ahead. It is not important to look up to the sky. Soften your jaw and relax your shoulders down your back.

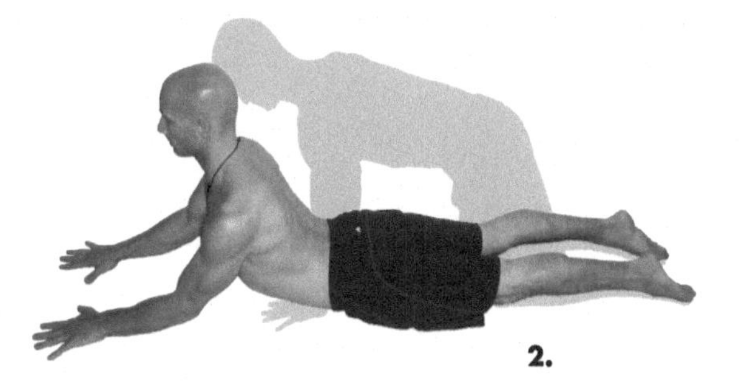

2.

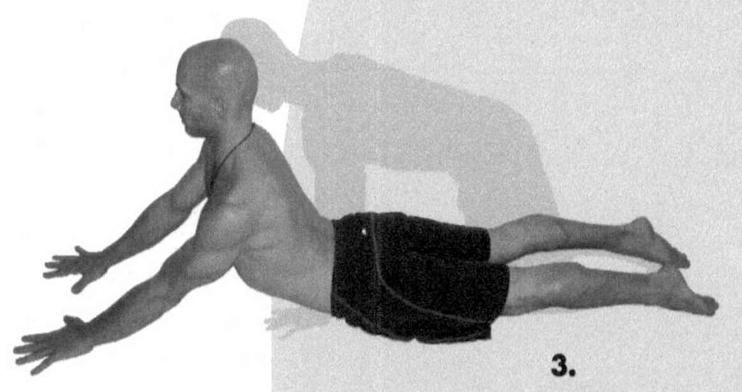

3.

SEATED TWIST • Rotation

Intention - To lubricate the joints of the mid and low back and decompress the mid and low back. To nourish the discs through imbibition (the process of bringing nutrients into the discs through specific movements).

Set Up: Begin Kneeling.

Movement:

1. Bring your left arm across the chest. Reach underneath with your right arm and cradle your elongated arm into a 90 degree angle.
Keep the top arm straight.

2. On the exhale, twist your torso to the right.
On the inhale, return to the center and repeat on the other side.

1. 2.

SIDE BEND • Lateral Flexion

Intention - To lubricate the joints of the mid and low back and open the side of the spine.

Set Up: Begin Kneeling.

Movement:

1. Clasp your hands behind the neck and extend your elbows out to the side.

2. On the exhale, bend sideways to the right.

KEYPOINT: Rather than crunching to the side, elongate upward as you bend to the side.

On the inhale, return to the center and repeat on the other side.

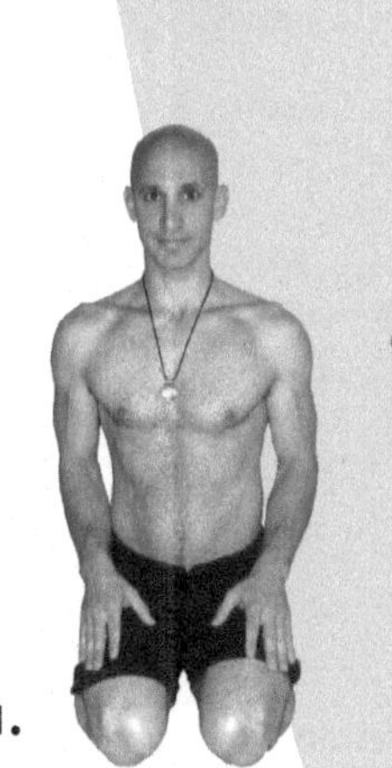

1.

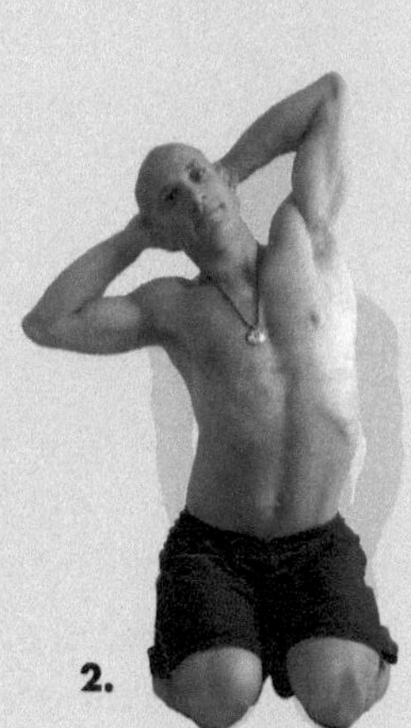

2.

BASIC MOVEMENTS OF THE LUMBAR SPINE

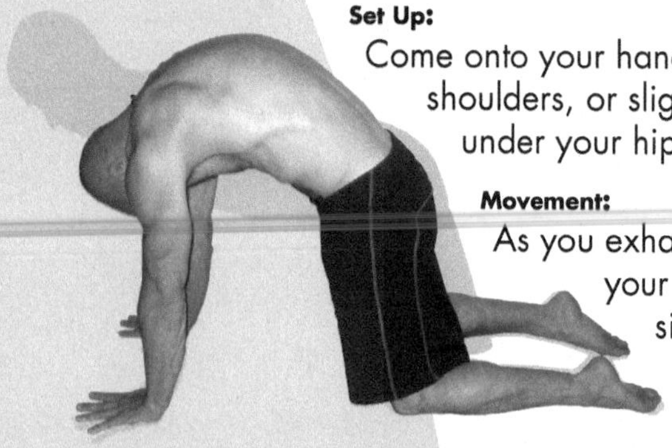

CAT TILT • Flexion of the Spine Posterior Rotation of the Pelvis

Intention - To lubricate the joints of the spine, the sacroiliac and hip. To nourish the discs through imbibition (the process of bringing nutrients into the discs through specific movements).

Set Up:

Come onto your hands and knees with your hands underneath your shoulders, or slightly in front of your shoulders. Position your knees under your hip bones.

Movement:

As you exhale, round your spine. Draw your navel in toward your spine, tuck your tail bone under. Point your sit bones toward the floor. Softly lower your chin to your chest.

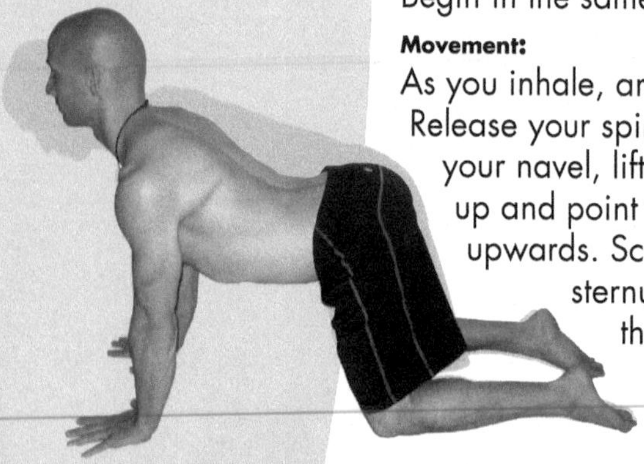

DOG TILT • Extension of the Spine Anterior Rotation of the Pelvis

Intention - To lubricate the joints of the spine, the sacroiliac and hip.
To nourish the discs through imbibition (the process of bringing nutrients into the discs through specific movements).

Set Up:

Begin in the same position as Cat Tilt.

Movement:

As you inhale, arch your spine. Release your spine down toward your navel, lift your tailbone up and point your sit bones upwards. Scoop your inner sternum up toward the sky.

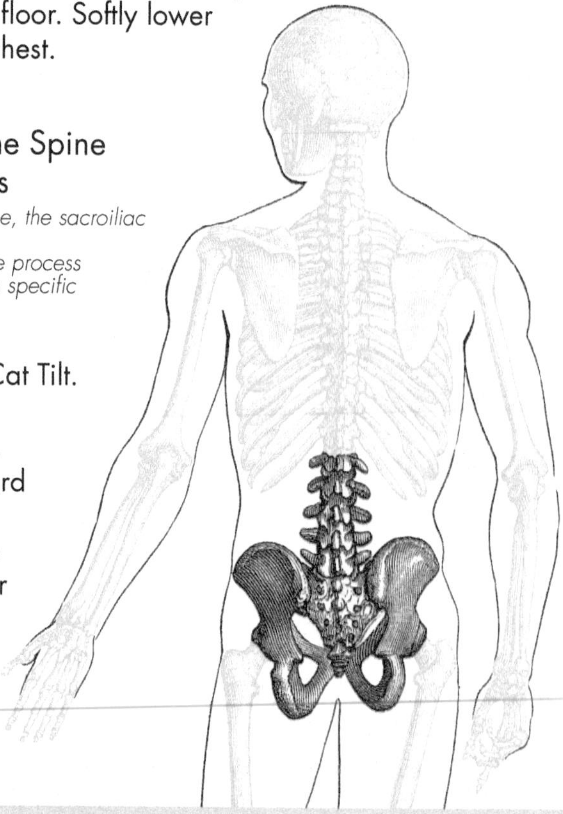

LUMBAR SPINE LUBRICATION • **"Root Down"**

Once you have unlocked your neck and expanded your heart center, you are ready to explore your power center.

This sequence of movements has been designed to "free up" the lower portion of your spine.

This region of your spine is responsible for how you connect with the earth. It relates to your structural and energetic foundation.

When your foundation is aligned, strong, and malleable, the organs and glands of digestion and reproduction, along with your muscles of locomotion can function at their highest level.

So when performing the movements of your low back remember to first pause.

Link each movement with your breath. With intense concentration you will activate the intelligence within your body and will achieve more advanced states of interconnectedness.

Remember to pause... relax deeply... breathe... and feel the effects.

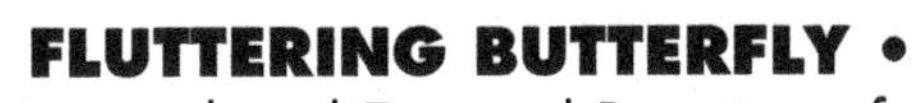

FLUTTERING BUTTERFLY • Internal and External Rotation of the Pelvis

Intention - To lubricate the hip and sacro iliac joints.

Set Up:

1. Lie on your back, with your feet flat on the floor.

Movement:

2. On the inhale, fan your knees apart and bring the soles of your feet together.

On the exhale, bring your knees back together.

3. On the inhale, bring your knees together and fan your feet apart.

Return to the center on the inhale and repeat.

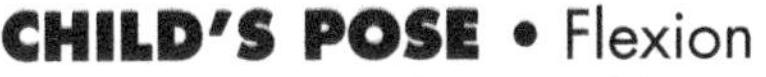

CHILD'S POSE • Flexion

Intention - To lubricate the joints of the spine, sacroiliac, and hips while in a rounded position. To gently traction the spine.

Set Up: Begin kneeling.

Movement: On the exhale, fold forward so that your chest lands softly on your thighs.

Extend your arms straight out in front of you. Look at your hands to make sure they are in line with your shoulders.

Anchor your hands into the floor by pressing the palms into the floor. Press into your hands to push your sit bones back onto your heels.

COBRA & SPHINX • Extension

Intention - To lubricate the joints of the mid and low back. To open the heart center and decompress the low back.

Set Up:

1. Lie on your stomach with your hands extended out in front of you.

Movement: On the inhale, press your hands gently into the floor, arch your spine, and lift your inner sternum toward the sky. *(See Variations **1** - **3**)*

KEYPOINT: Keep your head relaxed and looking straight ahead. It is not necessary to look up to the sky.
Soften your jaw and your shoulders.

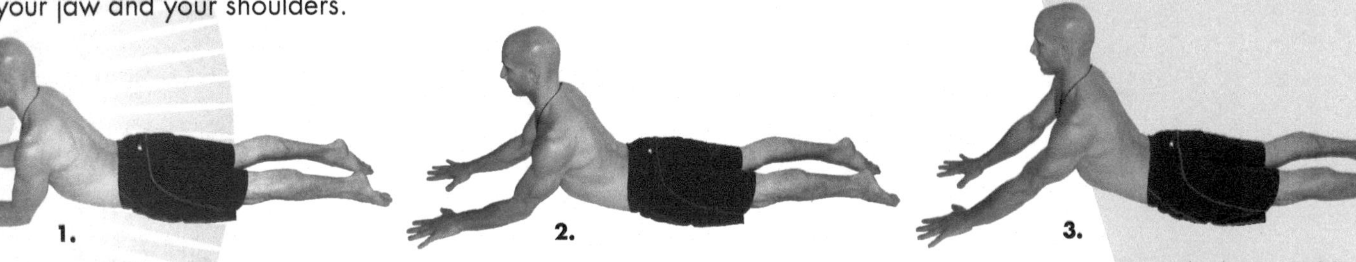

BASIC MOVEMENTS OF THE LUMBAR SPINE *(cont.)*

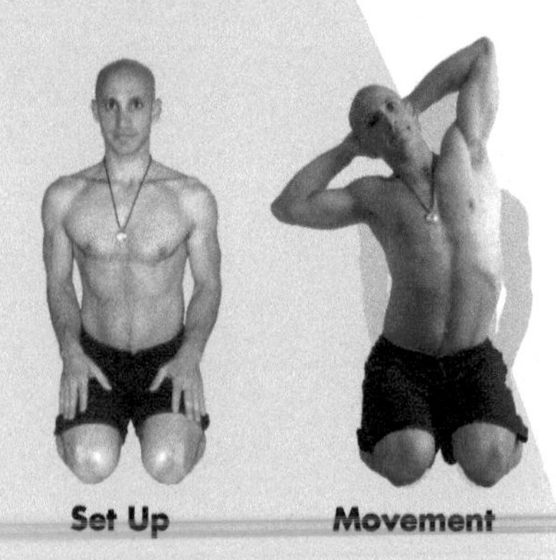

SIDE BEND • Lateral Flexion

Intention - To lubricate the joints of the mid and low back and open the side of the spine.

Set Up:
Clasp your hands behind the neck and extend your elbows out to the side.

Movement: On the exhale, bend sideways to the right.

KEYPOINT: Rather than crunching to the side, feel an elongation upward as you bend to the side.

On the inhale return to the center and repeat on the other side.

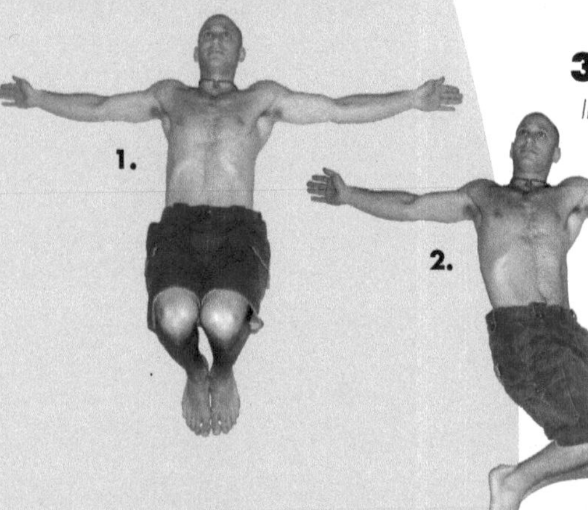

3 PART SPINAL TWIST • Rotation

Intention - To lubricate the joints of the sacro iliac and lumbar spine in sequential order.

Part 1: *Intention - To lubricate the joints of the hip and sacro iliac .*

1. Lie on your back, with your feet flat on the floor and your knees touching.

2. On the exhale, simply drop your knees over to the left, without changing your foot position.

On the inhale, return your knees back to the starting position and repeat on the other side.

Part 2: *Intention - To lubricate the joints of the sacro iliac and lower lumbar spine.*

Lie on your back, with your feet flat on the floor and your knees touching.

2. Raise your feet off the floor so that your shins and thighs make a pure 90 degree angle.

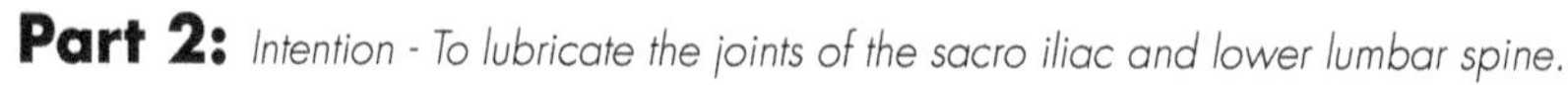

3. On the exhale, simply drop your knees over to the left, without changing your shin/thigh position.

On the inhale, return your knees back to the starting position and repeat on the other side.

Part 3: *Intention - To lubricate the joints of the middle and upper lumbar spine.*

Lie on your back, with your feet flat on the floor and your knees touching.

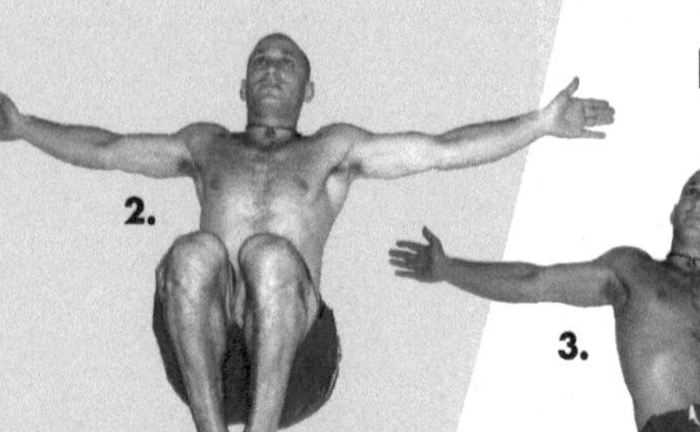

2. Raise your feet off the floor and bring your knees up as high as you can toward your chest.

3. On the exhale, simply drop your knees over to the left, without changing your knees/chest position.

On the inhale, return your knees back to the starting position and repeat on the other side.

BASIC TWISTS

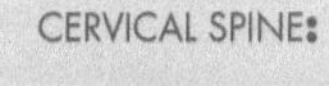
CERVICAL SPINE:

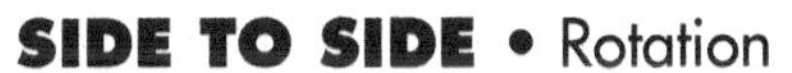

SIDE TO SIDE • Rotation

Intention - To lubricate, primarily, the joints between the top 2 vertebrae in the spine, the atlas and axis, as well as the rest of the cervical spine.

Movement:

On the exhale, while keeping your chin parallel to the floor, look over your right shoulder.
Return your head to center on the inhale and repeat to the left side.

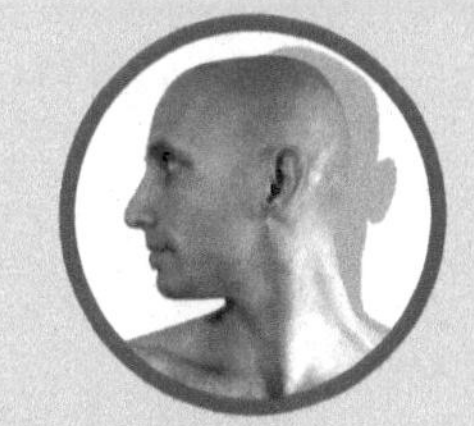

EAR TO SHOULDER • Lateral Flexion

Intention - Lubrication of all the joints of the neck.

Movement:

On the exhale, gently release your right ear to your right shoulder. On the inhale return your head to a neutral position.

KEYPOINT: Keep your shoulders relaxed and don't force the movement.

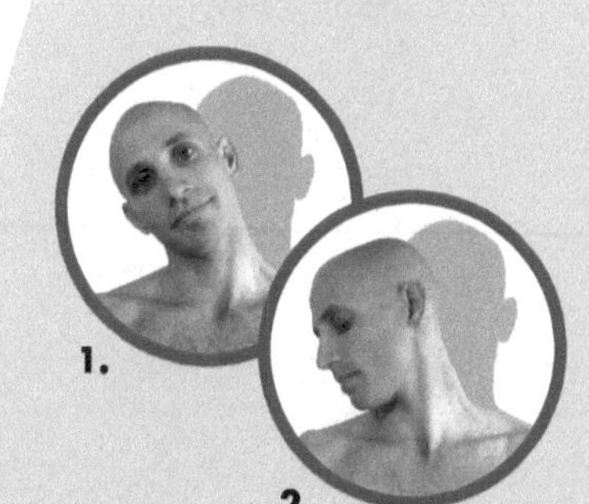

FUNKY CHICKEN PLUS FLEXION PLUS ROTATION

Intention - Lubrication of the joints at the top of the neck.

Movement:

1. Retract your chin backward.

2. Lower your chin toward your chest.

3a & 3b. Slowly rotate your chin to the left.

Return to the center and repeat to the right.

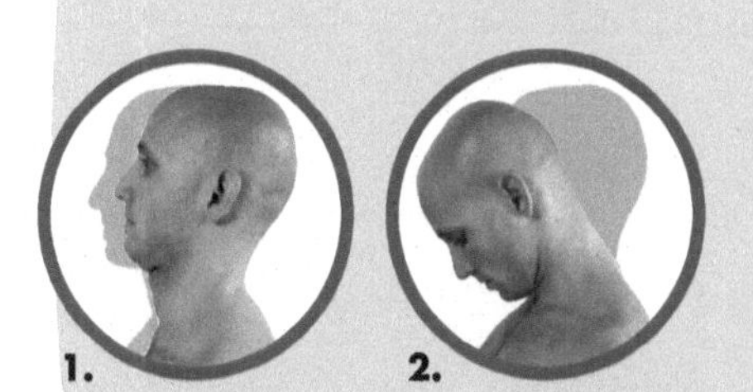

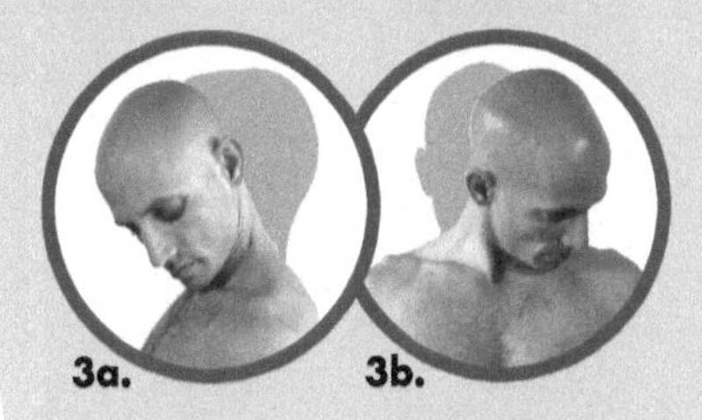

FUNKY CHICKEN PLUS EXTENSION PLUS ROTATION

Intention - Lubrication of the joints at the base of the neck and the top of the shoulders.

Movement:

1. Extend chin forward.

2. Raise your chin to the sky.

3a & 3b. Slowly rotate your chin to the left.

Return to the center and repeat to the right.

CAUTION: ***If you experience dizziness in this position, return your head to a straight forward position and sit down.***

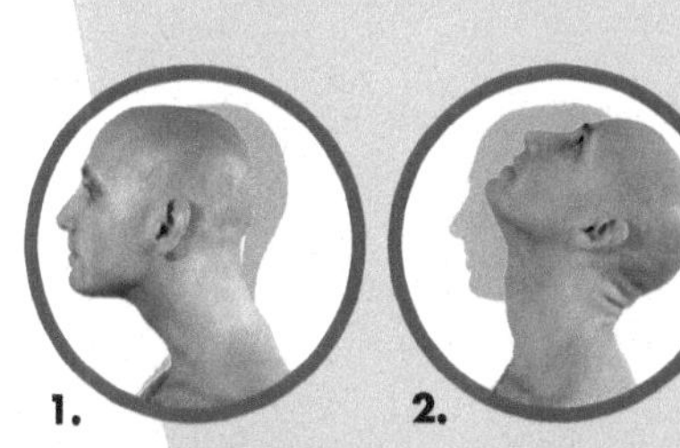

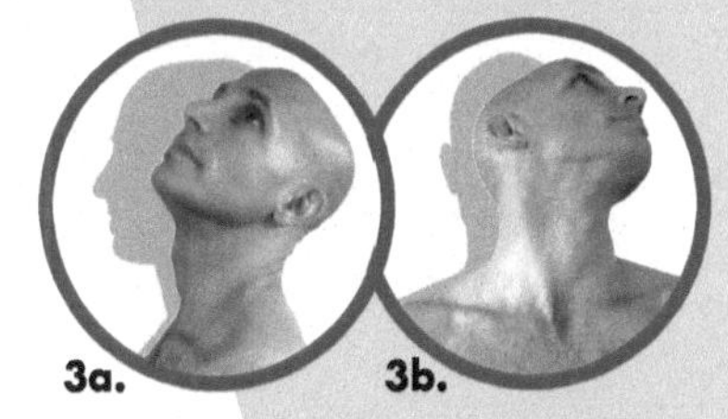

FULL SPINE LUBRICATION

"Twist It Out!"

Nothing feels better than a freely moveable spine.
So let's wring it out! This sequence is designed to unlock the rotational component of spinal movement.

Twists, according to the yogis of old, have the ability to energize and revitalize the body. So if you are in need of a "pick me up", insert this movement sequence into your normal routine and feel the effects.

Since we live in an industrialized society, we have lost the athletic ability to move like our Paleolithic ancestors. So as you do these movements, place your 'self' into the body of a 40,000-year-old hunter and gatherer, rolling around on the grassy plains and twisting under the sun.

Remember...
never force the movement...
breathe deeply...
move with respect...
and twist it out!

BASIC TWISTS - THORACIC SPINE *(cont.)*

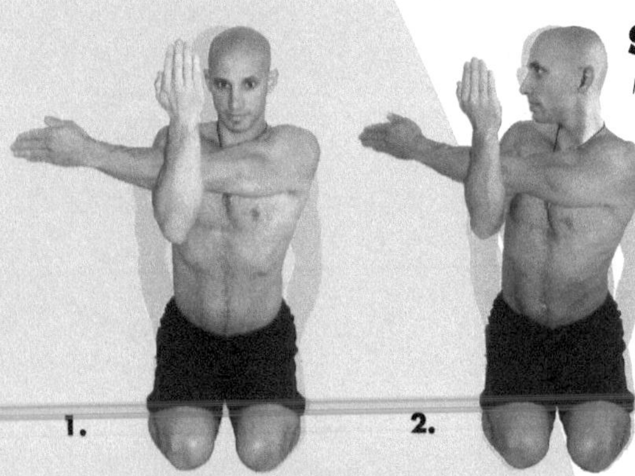

SEATED TWIST • Rotation

Intention - To lubricate the joints of the mid and low back and decompress the mid and low back. To nourish the discs through imbibition (the process of bringing nutrients into the discs through specific movements).

Set Up: Begin Kneeling.

Movement:

1. Bring your left arm across the chest. Reach underneath with your right arm and cradle your elongated arm into a 90 degree angle. Keep the top arm straight.

2. On the exhale twist your torso to the right. On the inhale return to the center and repeat on the other side.

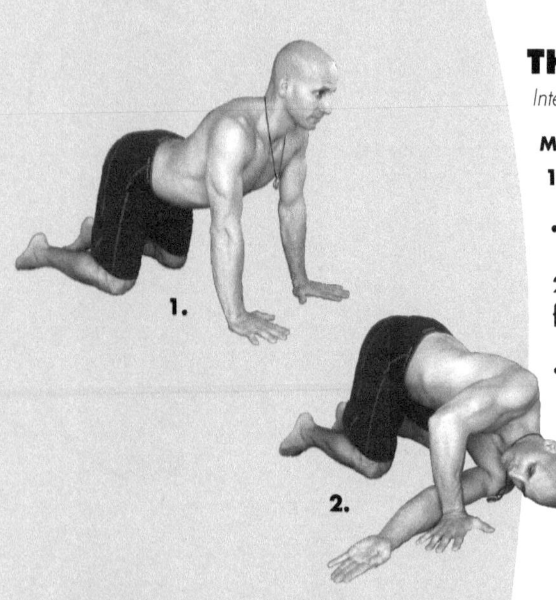

THREADING THE NEEDLE IN DOG TILT • Rotation

Intention - To twist the spine with emphasis on the lower to middle thoracic spine.

Movement:

1. Come onto your hands and knees.

• Arch your back and tilt your sit bones up.

2. Slide your left hand with palm facing up across your chest on the floor until your left shoulder gently touches the floor.

• Rotate your right hand so that both hands are facing the same direction. Press the right hand into the floor as you continue to tilt your sit bones up to the sky.

• Repeat on the other side.

BASIC TWISTS - LUMBAR SPINE

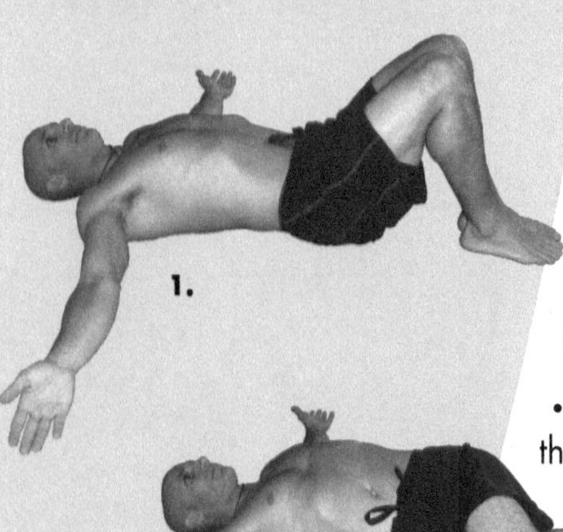

5 PART SPINAL TWIST • Rotation

Intention - To lubricate the joints of the sacro iliac and lumbar spine in sequential order.

Part 1: *Intention - To lubricate the joints of the hip and sacro iliac .*

1. Lie on your back with your feet flat on the floor and your knees touching.

2. On the exhale, simply drop your knees over to the left, without changing your foot position.

• On the inhale, return your knees back to the starting position and repeat on the other side.

5 PART SPINAL TWIST • Continued

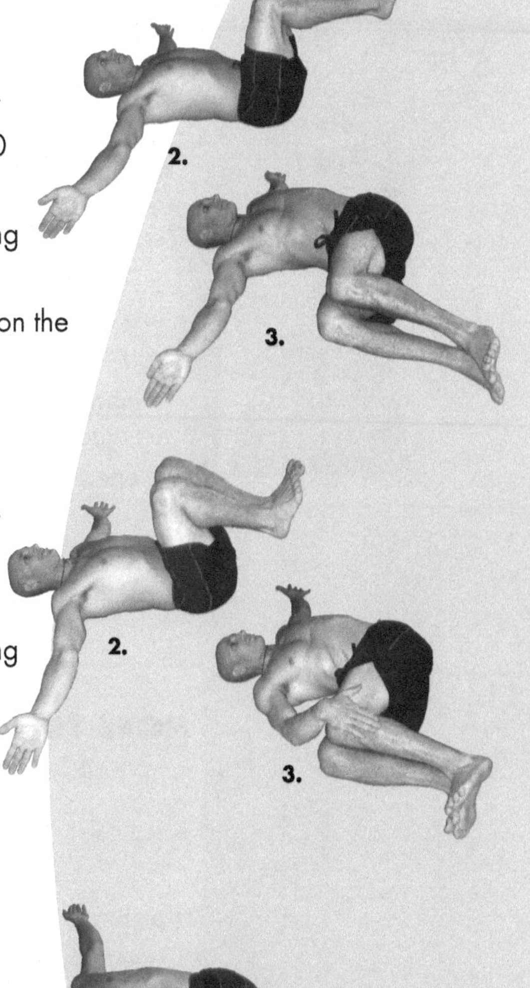

Part 2: *Intention - To lubricate the joints of the sacro iliac and lower lumbar spine.*

• Lie on your back, with your feet flat on the floor and your knees touching.

2. Raise your feet off the floor so that your shins and thighs make a pure 90 degree angle.

3. On the exhale, simply drop your knees over to the right, without changing your shin/thigh position.

• On the inhale, return your knees back to the starting position and repeat on the other side.

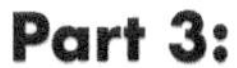

Part 3:

Intention - To lubricate the joints of the middle and upper lumbar spine.

• Lie on your back, with your feet flat on the floor and your knees touching.

2. Raise your feet off the floor and bring your knees up as high as you can toward your chest.

3. On the exhale, simply drop your knees over to the right, without changing your knees/ chest position.

• On the inhale, return your knees back to the starting position and repeat on the other side.

Part 4:

Intention - To lubricate the joints of the middle and upper lumbar spine.

• Lie on your back, with both legs straight out on the floor.

• Bring your left knee into the chest. Maintain an arch in the lower back.

• On the exhale, drop your bent right knee over to the left.

• On the inhale, return your knees to the starting position.
Repeat on the other side.

Part 5: Spinal Twist with Strap and Straight Leg:

Intention - To lubricate the joints of the middle and upper lumbar spine.

• Lie on your back with your feet flat on the floor.

2. Wrap a strap around your right foot and straighten your knee.

3. On the exhale, drop your straight right leg over to the left.
Keep your left knee bent while maintaining an arch in the lower back.

• On the inhale, return your knees to the starting position.
Repeat on the other side.

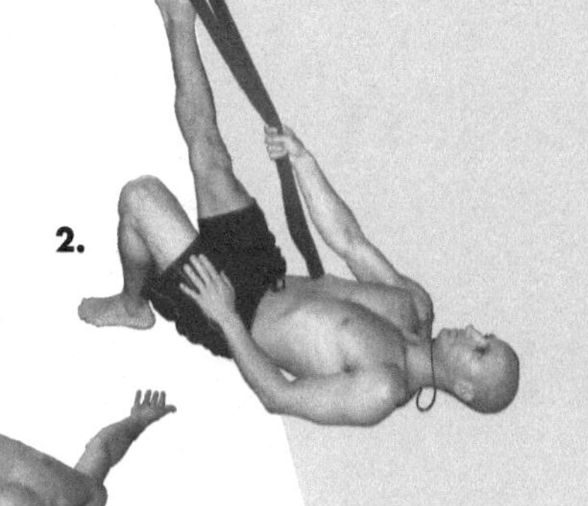

3.

BASIC STRETCHES FOR THE NECK

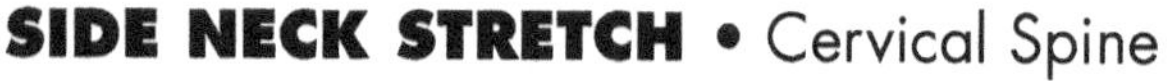

SIDE NECK STRETCH • Cervical Spine

Intention: To stretch the side muscles of the neck.

Stretch:

- Center yourself by lifting your inner sternum up and neutralize your head.
- Exhale, and gently release your right ear to your right shoulder.
- Take your right hand and gently rest it over your left ear.
- Let it settle.
- Inhale, and return your head to the starting position.
- Repeat on the other side.

Gem: *Keep your shoulders relaxed and don't force the movement. Be kind to your spine. Let gravity do its thing.*

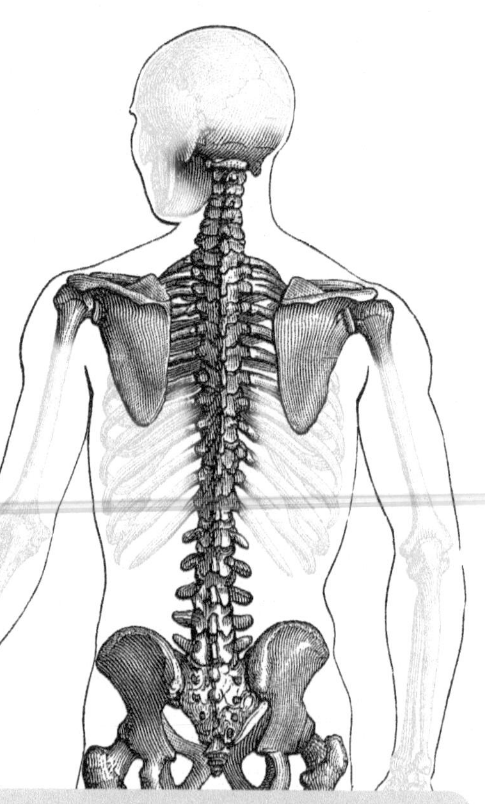

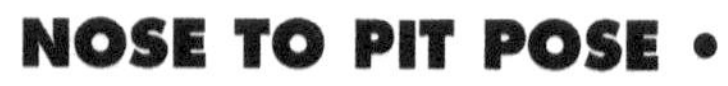

NOSE TO PIT POSE • Cervical Spine

Intention:

To stretch the side and back muscles of the neck.

Stretch:

- Center yourself by lifting your inner sternum up and neutralize your head.
- Exhale, and gently release your right ear to your right shoulder.
- Rotate your nose until it is angled toward your arm pit.
- Take your right hand and gently rest it over the back of your skull.
- Let it settle.
- Inhale, and return your head to the starting position.
- Repeat on the other side.

Gem: *Keep your shoulders relaxed and don't force the movement.*
Be kind to your spine. Let gravity do its thing.

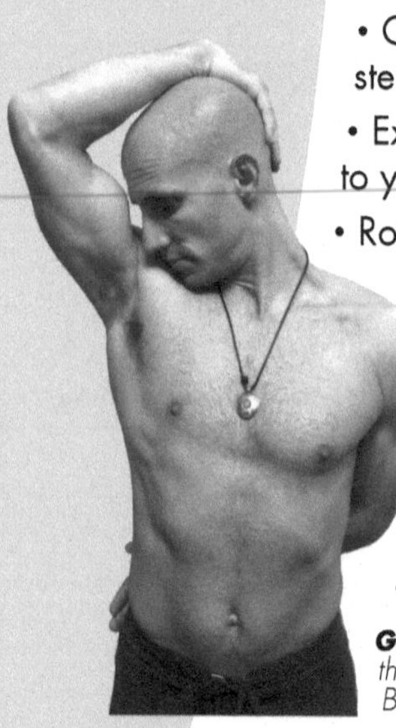

MUSCLE ELONGATION

"Stretch It Out!"

Motion is life! And when the muscles of the spine are able to expand and contract naturally, your body becomes more energy efficient.

Stretching your muscles allows them to be free from spasmodic contractions and fibrotic adhesions.

Stretch to improve energy levels and decrease your risk of injury. Do it upon rising, at lunch, and before you go to bed for maximum results.

Practice this ancient form of exercise to get the most from your body. Do it slowly, don't force it.

Breathe into the stretch, and then feel the effects.

Mountain Pose: Begin most stretches in this position to find your center.

BASIC STRETCHES FOR THE NECK *(cont.)*

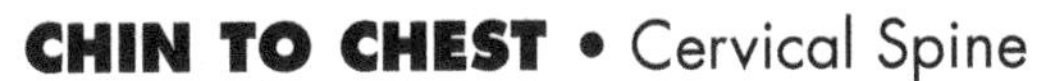

CHIN TO CHEST • Cervical Spine

Intention: To stretch the side and back muscles of the neck.

Stretch:

- Center yourself by lifting your inner sternum up and neutralizing your head.
- Exhale, and gently release your head forward.
- Take both hands to the back of your skull and let the weight of your hands provide the stretch.
- Let it settle.
- Inhale, and return your head to the starting position.
- Perform the cervical spine movement sequence to recalibrate the neck, and its muscles and joints.

Gem: *Keep your shoulders relaxed and don't force the movement. Let gravity do its thing. Be kind to your spine.*

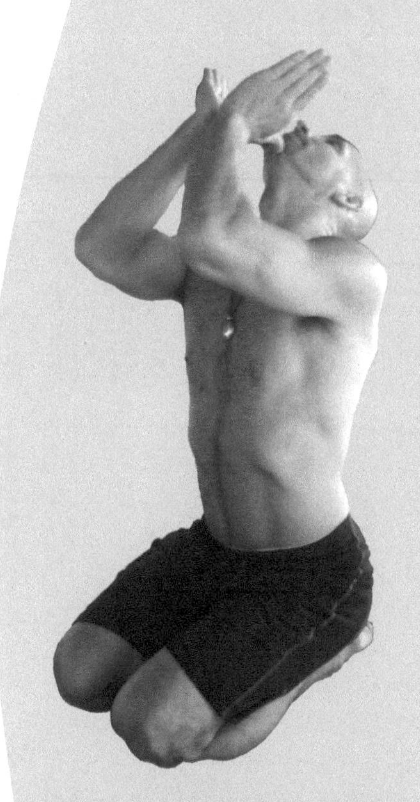

CHIN TO SKY • Cervical Spine

Intention: To stretch the front side muscles of the neck and promote a healthy cervical curve.

- Center yourself by lifting your inner sternum up and neutralize your head.
- Gently glide your chin forward and extend your head backward.
- Take the tips of your thumbs and lightly push upward.
- Breathe comfortably.
- Exhale, and return your head to the starting position.
- Perform the cervical spine movement sequences to recalibrate the neck and its muscles and joints.

NOTE: ***If you experience dizziness in this position, return your head to a straight forward position and sit down.***

BASIC STRETCHES FOR THE SHOULDERS

ARM PRETZEL • Cervical Spine & Shoulder

Intention: To stretch the deltoids/shoulders and the rhomboids (the muscles in-between your shoulder blades).

Stretch:

- Center yourself by lifting your inner sternum up and neutralizing your head.

1. Bring your right arm across the chest

- Reach underneath with your left arm and cradle your elongated arm into a 90 degree angle.
- Keep the top arm straight.

2. Bend your right elbow and connect your palms.

- Breathe in-between your shoulder blades.
- Let it settle.
- Release, return to the center, and then repeat on the other side.

1.

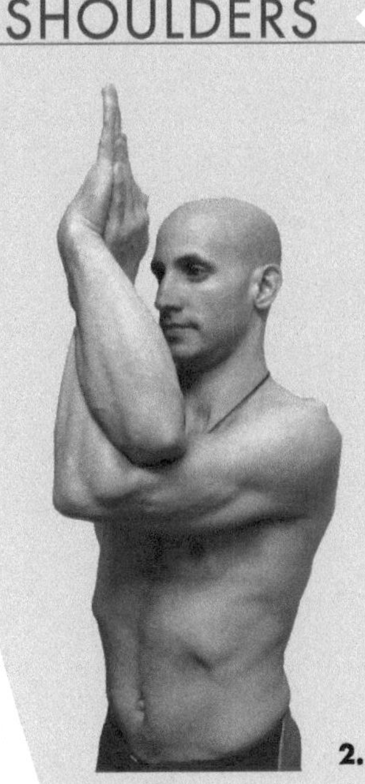

2.

BASIC STRETCHES FOR THE SHOULDERS *(cont.)*

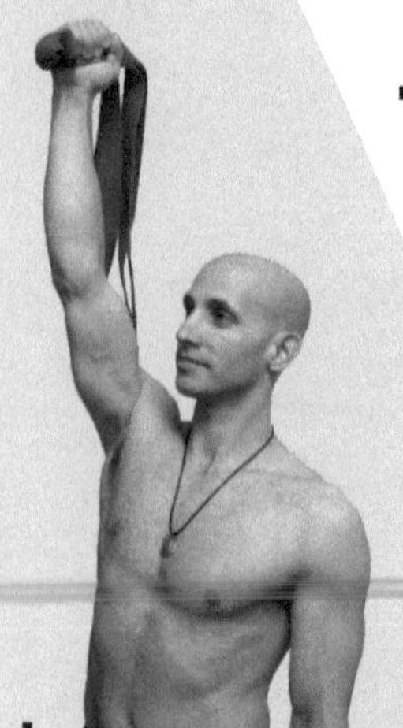

1.

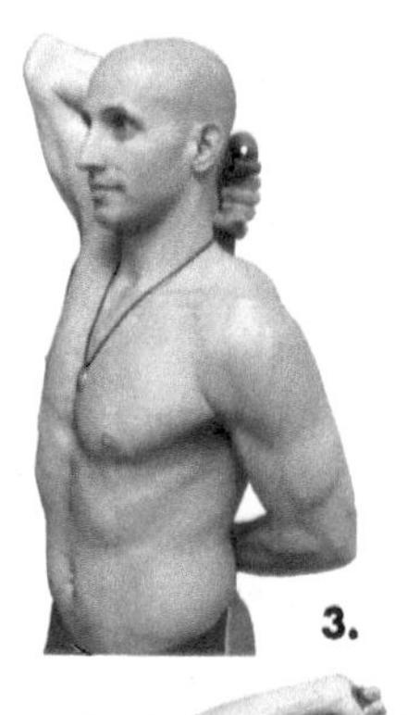

3.

THE UP & UNDER • Cervical Spine & Shoulder

Intention: To stretch the triceps, upper latisimus dorsi, and the external rotators of the shoulder.

Stretch:

- Center yourself.

1. Hold a towel in your right hand.

- Inhale and raise your right arm straight up with your palm facing your face.

2. Exhale, bend your right elbow.

- Clasp your right elbow with your left hand and gently move your right elbow backward...slowly.

3. Release your right elbow and bring your left hand behind your back.

- Grab the towel and gently pull downward.

4. Then, reverse the direction and pull up ...slowly... to get a stretch on the bottom arm.

- Release, shake out your arms, and then repeat on the other side.

Gem: *Keep your inner sternum lifted and your lower ribs moving down toward the floor.*

2.

4.

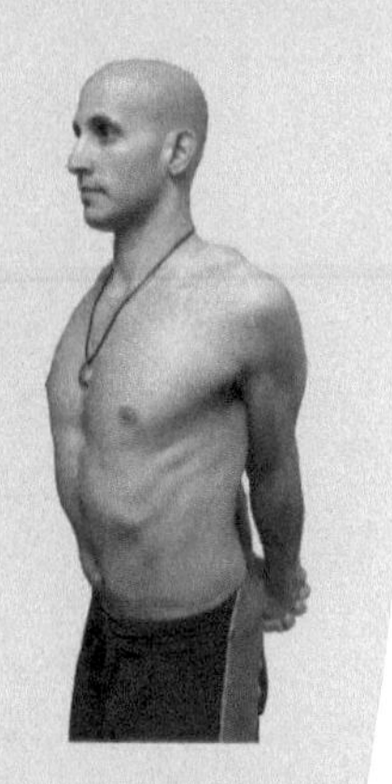

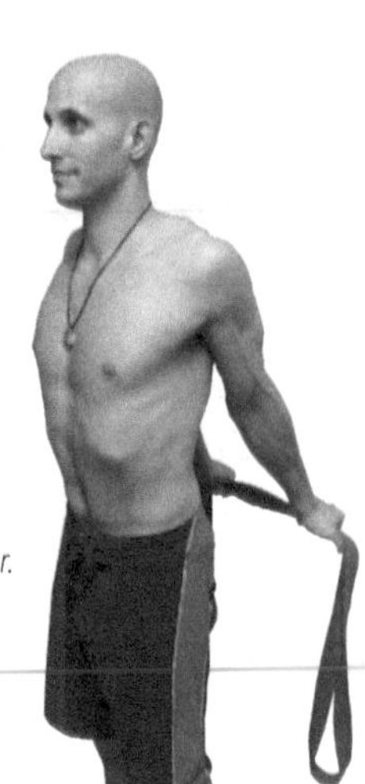

CHEST EXPANSION STRETCH • Shoulders

Intention: To stretch the chest/pectoralis and the biceps.

Stretch:

- Center yourself.
- Reach your hands behind your back and clasp your hands.
- Inhale, and gently raise your arms behind your back.
- Let it settle.
- Release, and shake out your arms.

Gem: *Keep your inner sternum lifted and your lower ribs moving down toward the floor.*

BASIC STRETCHES FOR THE HIPS & LEGS

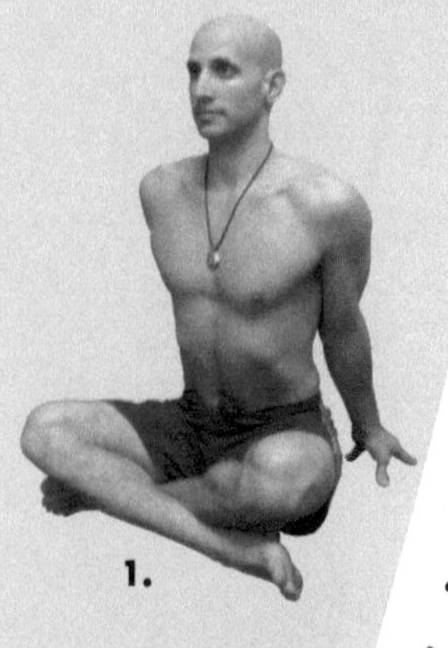

1.

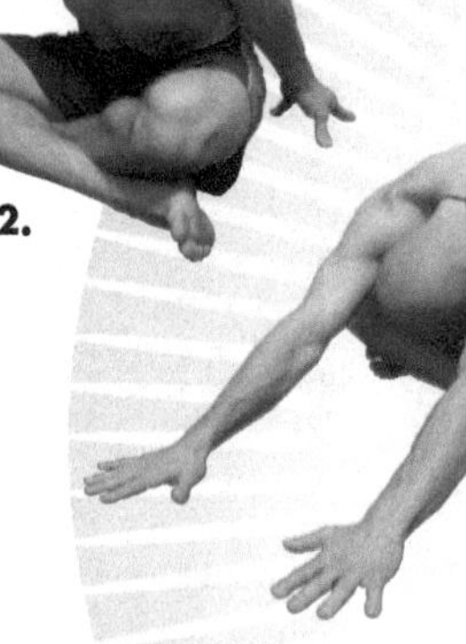

2.

EASY CROSS-LEGGED POSE • Hips

Intention: To stretch the adductors and internal rotators of the hips.

Stretch:

- Center yourself.

1. Cross your right leg in front of your left.
Move toward getting your heels under your knees.

2. Exhale, and bend forward from your hips while keeping your spine straight.

3. Then slowly let the back round.

- Let it settle.
- Inhale, and return to a seated upright position.
- Repeat on the other side.

Gem: *Sit up as straight as possible.*

DIAMOND POSE • Hips

Intention: To stretch the adductors and internal rotators of the hips.

Stretch:

- Center yourself.
1. Position your feet in a diamond position.
2. Exhale, and bend forward from your hips while keeping your spine straight.
   - Then slowly let the back round.
   - Let it settle.
- Inhale, and return to an upright-seated diamond position.
- Repeat on the other side.

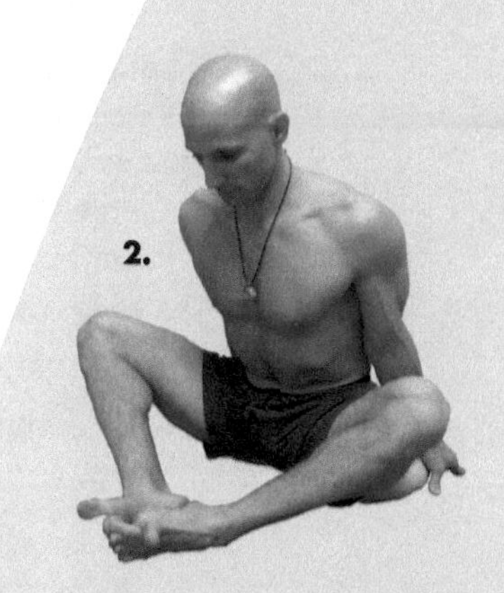

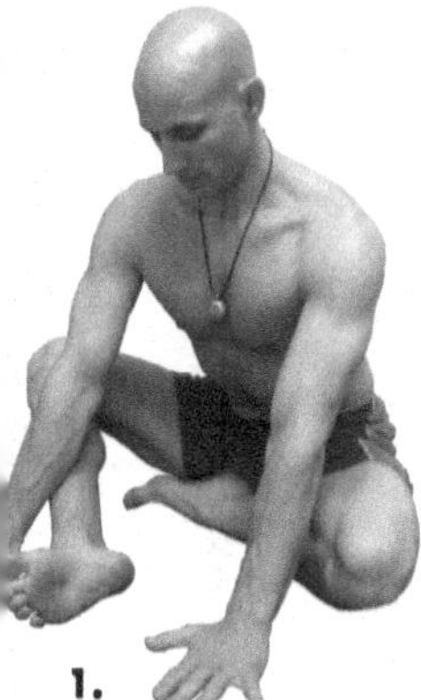

HALF DIAMOND POSE • Hips

Intention: To stretch the adductors and internal rotators of the hips.

Stretch:

- Center yourself.
- Position your feet in a diamond position.
1. Bring your left foot in toward your pubic bone, while keeping your right foot in the same place.
2. Exhale, and bend forward from your hips while keeping your spine straight.
- Then slowly let the back round.
- Let it settle.
- Inhale, and return to an upright-seated half diamond position.
- Repeat on the other side.

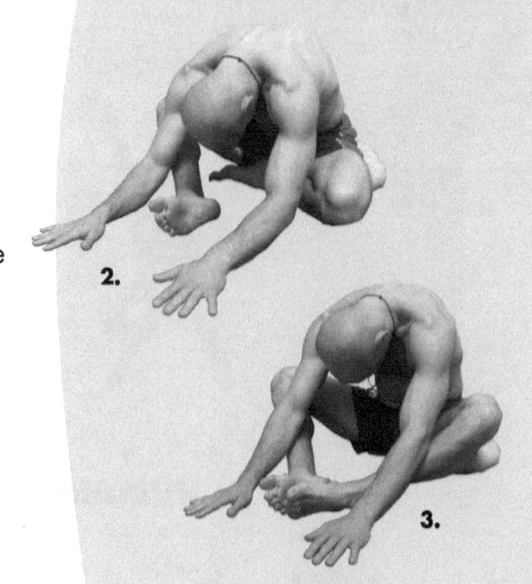

LOVE MY HIPS POSE • Hips

Intention: To stretch the abductors and rotators of the hips.

Stretch:

- Center yourself.
- Beginning in Easy Cross Legged Pose, cross your right foot over your left thigh.
- As you hug your right knee into your spine, press your sit bones into the floor, inhale, and extend your spine straight up.
- Let it settle.
- Repeat on the other side.

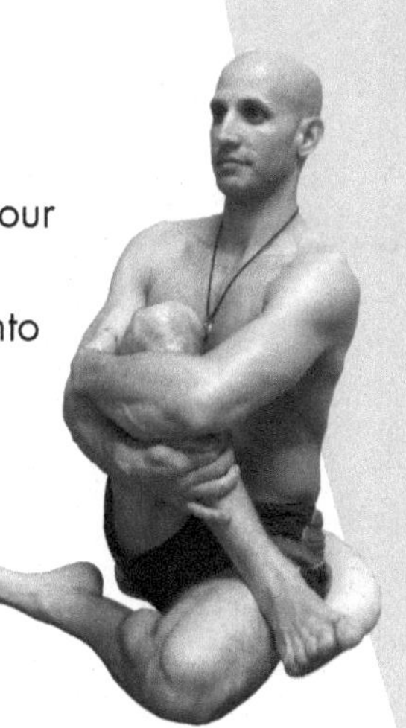

ATLAS KNEELING POSE • Hips

Intention: To stretch the quadriceps and hips.

Stretch:

- Center yourself.
- From Samurai/Lightning Bolt Pose, step your right foot forward until your right knee is over your right ankle.
- Exhale, and engage your entire body forward to deepen the stretch.
- Return to Samurai/Lightning Bolt Pose and repeat on the other side.

Gem: *Keep hips in line with one another. Press firmly into the top of your back foot to maintain your balance.*
Also feel free to incorporate all shoulder stretches in this position.

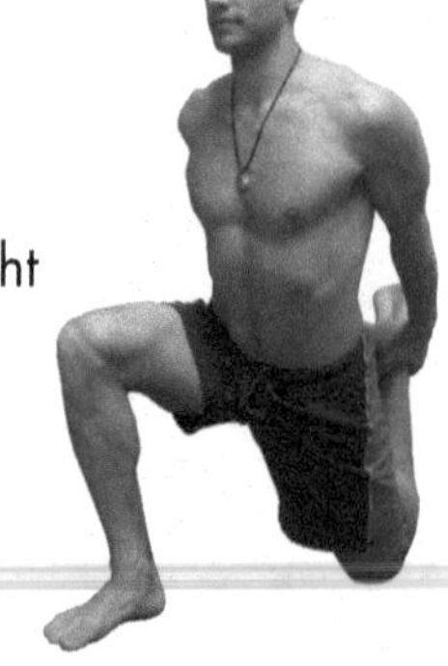

STANDING HAMSTRING

Intention: To stretch the hamstrings.

Stretch:

- Find your center in Mountain Pose.

1. Place your right foot on a surface in front of you.

2. Exhale, and bend forward from your hips while keeping your spine straight.

- Inhale, and return to an upright position.
- Repeat on the other side.

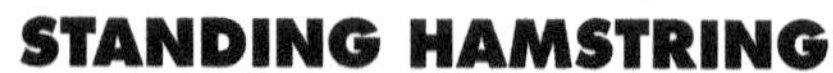

Gem: *Keep hips in line with one another. Draw up your kneecap on both thighs by contracting your quadriceps muscle. Do not round your back or force the stretch.*

1.

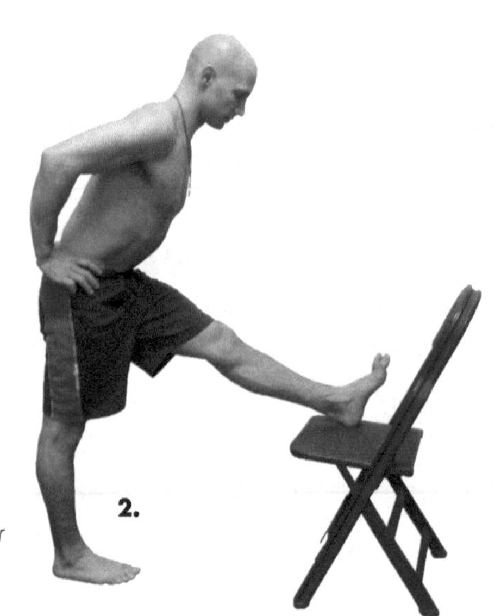

2.

HUMAN "L" & "V" POSE

Intention: To stretch the hamstrings and adductors.

Stretch:

1. Lie on your back with your feet up the wall in an "L" position. Let it settle.

2. Exhale, and open your legs wide apart.

Gem: *Keep your low back on the floor. You may have to inch back away from the wall to achieve this position.*

1.

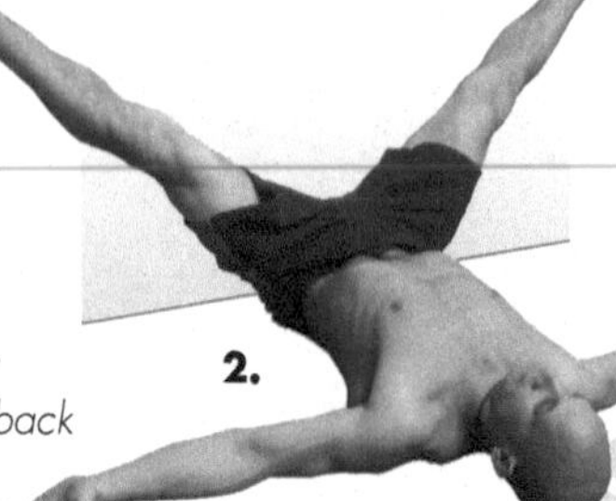

2.

FIGURE 4 POSE • Hips

Intention: To stretch the internal rotators of the hip.

Stretch:

- Lie on your back with your thighs and legs forming a ninety degree angle.
- Exhale, and place your right ankle above your left knee.
- Let it settle.
- Repeat on the other side.

Gem: *Keep your low back on the floor. You may have to inch back away from the wall to achieve this position.*

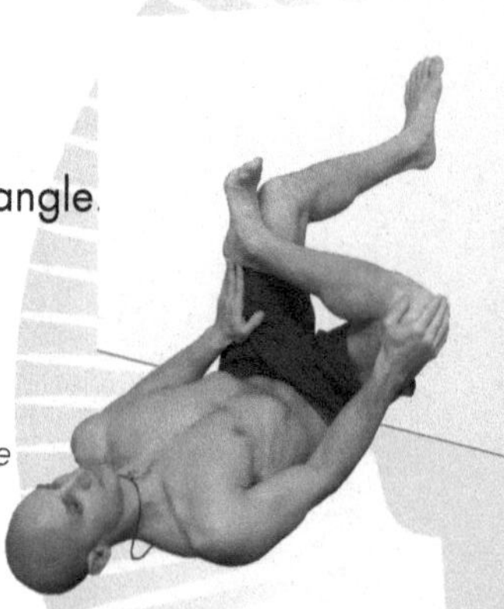

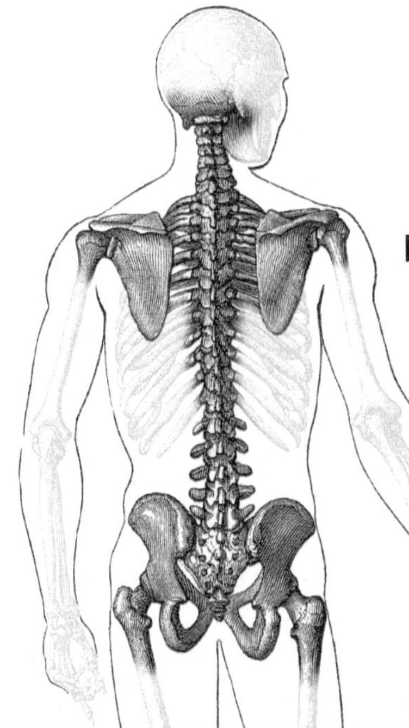

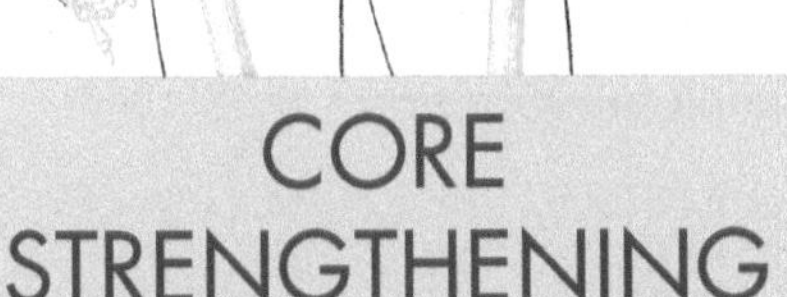

CORE STRENGTHENING

"Hard Core!"

So what is optimal alignment?
It is a state in which the architecture of the body is positioned in such a way that balances gravity, promotes a healthy distribution of weight, encourages full range of motion based on the body's natural design, and allows for maximum expression of the nervous system without interference.

With a powerful core that stretches from the top of the head to the bottom of the spine, optimal alignment is solidified and maintained.

Misalignment is reduced through correct form, proper movement, intelligent stretching and strengthening, which all help power up the body's energy system.

We strengthen our core so that we are able to stand tall against the effects of gravity and daily stress. So that they won't impede with life force.

In our daily life we give supreme attention to the core to hold the body upright, maintaining your energy.

With impeccable alignment and skillful movement, and a powerful core you are able to walk on this planet with powerful conviction!

RESISTED REVERSE FUNKY CHICKEN • Cervical Spine

Intention:
To strengthen the posterior/back muscles of the neck.

Strengthen:

- Lie on your back.
- With your chin level, gently press your head directly back into the floor.
- Hold for several breaths and then release.
- Repeat three to five times.

Gem:
Do not force the movement. If you feel pain, back off and apply less pressure. If pain persists, stop.

CRUNCH • Abdominals

Intention:
To strengthen the abdominals.

Strengthen:

1. Lie on your back and place your hands behind your head.

- Bend your knees to form ninety degree angle with your torso.

2. Exhale, and slowly contract your abdomen by bringing your chest toward your knees.

- Inhale, and slowly lower back down.
- Repeat as many times as possible while maintaining good form.

Gem: *Do not force your neck.*

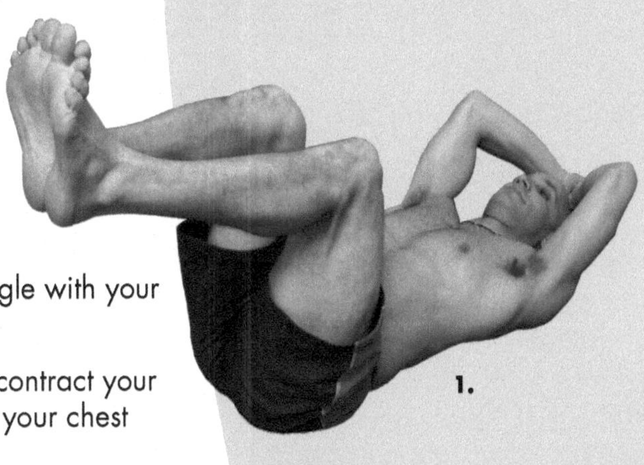

1.

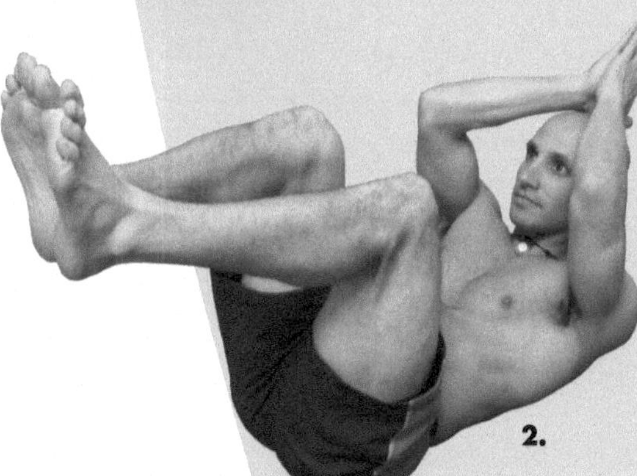

2.

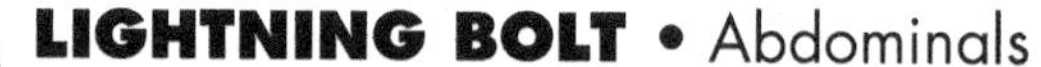

LIGHTNING BOLT • Abdominals

Intention: To strengthen the abdominals.

Strengthen:

- Lie on your back and place your hands by your side.
- Bend your knees to form ninety degree angle with your torso.
- Lift your upper back off the floor and maintain a crunch.
- Exhale, and slowly bring your right knee in toward your right shoulder, while straightening your left leg.
- Pause and inhale.
- Exhale and switch sides.
- Repeat as many times as possible while maintaining good form.

Gem: *Keep your spine in a flexed position at all times without arching the low back.*

TWISTING BOLTS • Abdominals

Intention: *To strengthen the abdominals and obliques*

Strengthen:

- Lie on your back and place your hands behind your head.
- Bend your knees to form ninety degree angle with your torso.
- Lift your upper back off the floor and maintain the crunch.
- Exhale, and slowly bring your right knee in toward your right shoulder, while twisting your torso to approximate your left elbow to the right knee.
- Pause and inhale.
- Exhale, and switch sides.
- Repeat as many times as possible while maintaining good form.

Gem: *Keep your spine in a flexed position at all times without arching the low back.*

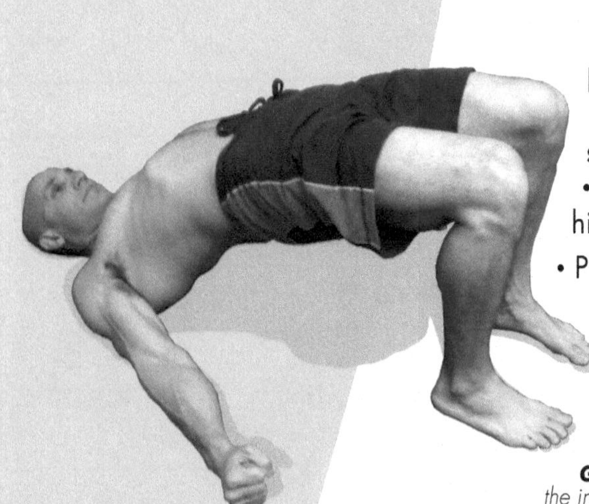

PELVIC LIFTS • Pelvic Floor

Intention: *To strengthen the floor of the pelvis.*

Strengthen:

- Lie on your back with your knees bent and your feet flat on the floor, hips width apart.
- Press your outer arms into the floor as you inhale, and lift your pelvis off the floor.
- Hold for a few breaths, then exhale and release down.
- Switch and repeat as many times as possible, while maintaining good form.

Gem: *Keep your knees from falling away from the starting position. Place a block in between the inner thighs to prevent this from happening. Keep your chin in a neutral position and avoid tucking your chin.*

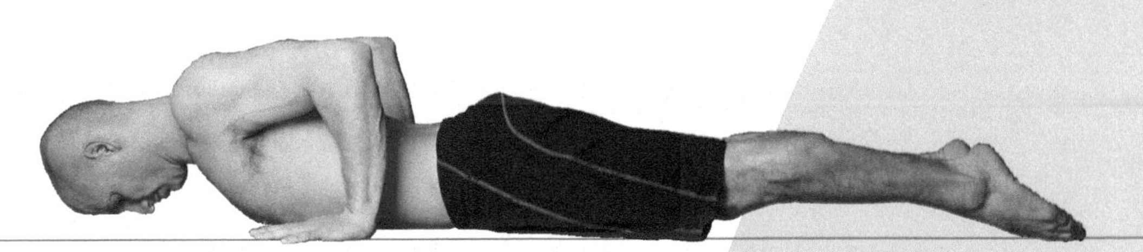

COBRA #1 • Dorsal Spine Strengtheners

Intention: *To strengthen the erector spinale muscles.*

Strengthen:

- Lie on your belly and place your hands by your side.
- Keep your gaze down.
- Inhale and lift your chest off the floor.
- Exhale, and release down.
- Repeat as many times as possible while maintaining good form.

Gem: *Keep your neck relaxed.*

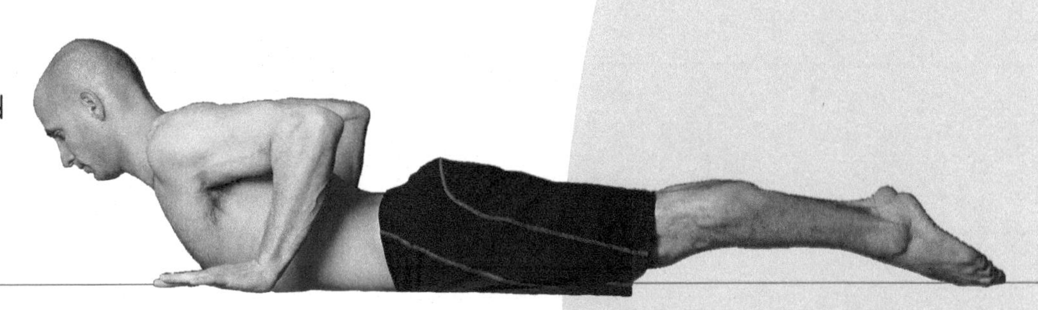

COBRA #2

Strengthen:

- This time keep your hands on the floor and lift your legs off the floor.
- Lengthen your tailbone toward the floor as you extend your legs.
- Roll your inner thighs up toward the sky and extend through the toes.
- Gaze straight ahead and breathe freely.

Gem: *Keep your neck relaxed.*

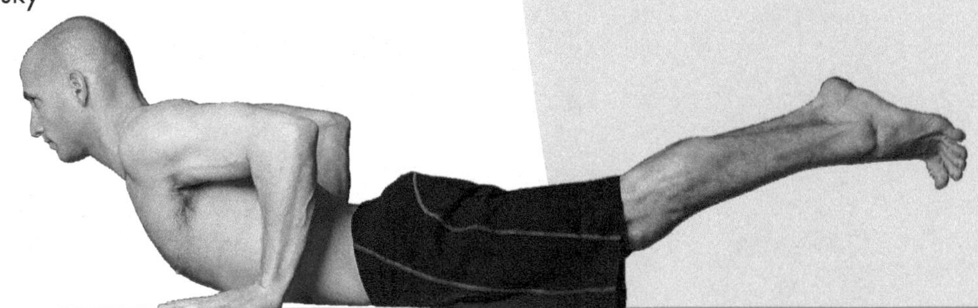

COBRA #3

Strengthen:

- Inhale, lift your hands and legs off the floor.
- Gaze straight ahead.
- Breathe comfortably and naturally.

Gem: *Keep your neck relaxed.*

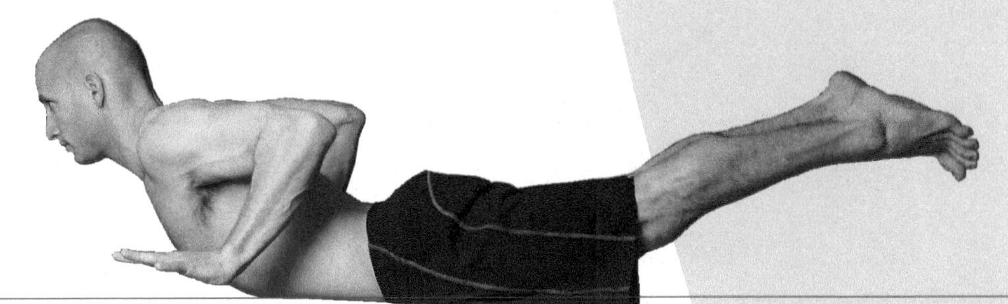

ALL 4'S- ALTERNATING LEGS & ARMS

• Dorsal Spine Strengtheners

Intention: *To strengthen the erector spinale muscles*

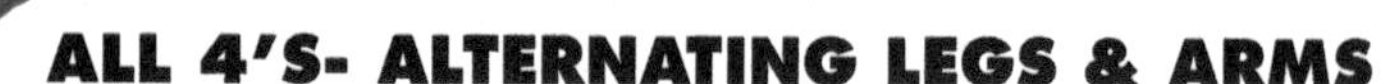

Strengthen:

- Come onto all fours.
- Keep your eye gaze looking down.
- Find your core by contracting your upper abs into the body and releasing your tailbone downward.
- Inhale and lift your right hand off the floor and extend it next to your head, while lifting and extending your left thigh and leg backward.
- Hold for a few breaths and then exhale and release down.
- Switch and repeat as many times as possible while maintaining good form.

Gem: *Try to maintain a neutral spine and minimize over-arching.*

KEGELS • Pelvic Floor

Intention: *To strengthen the floor of the pelvis*

Strengthen:

- Sit in Samurai Pose.
- Imagine that you're trying to stop yourself from passing gas and trying to stop the flow of urine midstream at the same time.
- The feeling is one of "squeeze and lift".
- Hold each Kegel for eight to ten seconds before releasing, and relax for a few seconds after each one.

Gem: *Make sure that you're squeezing and lifting without pulling in your tummy, squeezing your legs together, tightening your buttocks, or holding your breath.*

CORPSE POSE

It is no secret that the major premise of chiropractic focuses on the restoration and preservation of one's health, healing, and vitality. Ironically, Corpse Pose is one of the most powerful asanas that one can use to reenergize.

"Corpse Pose", alternately spelled Shavasana or Savasana, is often used to begin and to conclude a yoga session. It is a relaxing posture intended to rejuvenate one's body-mind.

How to:
Lying on your back, spread your arms and legs about 45 degrees from the sides of your body. Tilt head slightly back so it rests comfortably. Make sure you are warm and comfortable.

Close the eyes, and start by deepening the breath using full spine breathing. Allow your whole body to relax and merge with the earth. As the body relaxes, feel the whole body rising and falling with each breath.

Scan the body from toes to fingers, to the crown of the head, looking for tension, tightness and contracted muscles.

Consciously release and relax any pockets of tension you find. If you need to, rock or wiggle that part of your body from side to side.

Sometimes we need to experience life as a corpse to feel just how alive we are!

Release all control of the breath, the mind, and the body. Let your body move deeper and deeper into a state of total relaxation.

Relax the skin of the forehead, especially around the bridge of the nose between the eyebrows. Let the eyes sink to the back of the head, then turn them downward to gaze at the heart. Drop your brain to the back of the head.

Stay in savasana for 5 to 15 minutes.

Connect the energy field around your body.

To release:
Slowly deepen the breath, wiggle the fingers and toes, reach the arms over the head and stretch the whole body. Exhale, bend the knees into the chest, and roll to one side, preferably the right, coming into a fetal position. When you are ready, slowly inhale your way up to a seated position, moving your head slowly after. The head should always come up last.

You may notice that you see, hear, smell, and taste life differently after this pose.

Notes:
While savasana is a good way to reduce stress and tension, it is not recommended for meditation as it has a tendency to induce sleepiness.

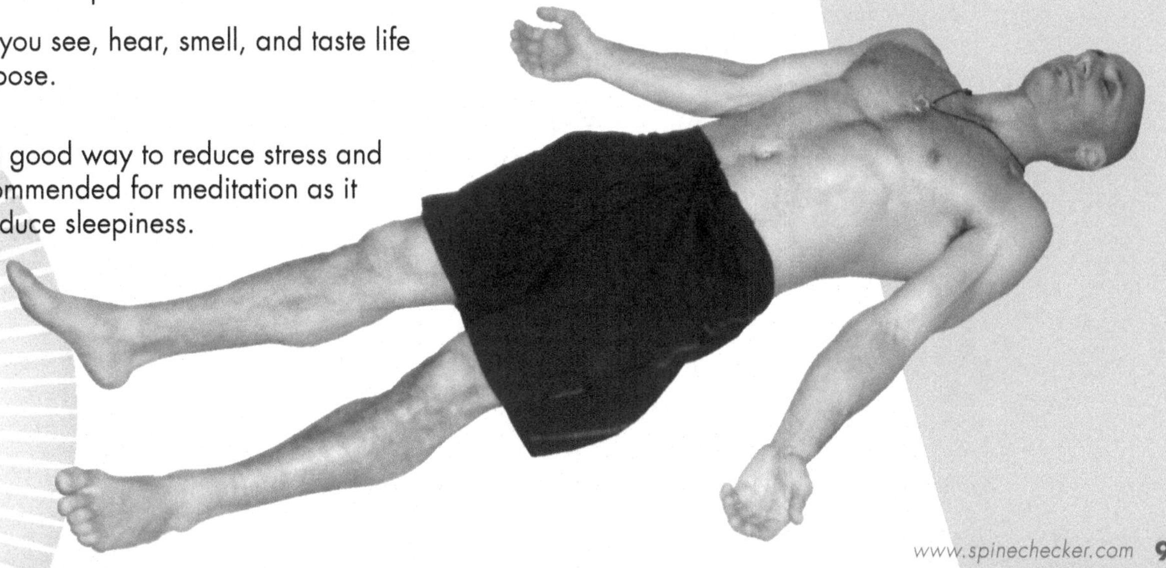

BREATHING, CONCENTRATION, MEDITATION & AFFIRMATIONS

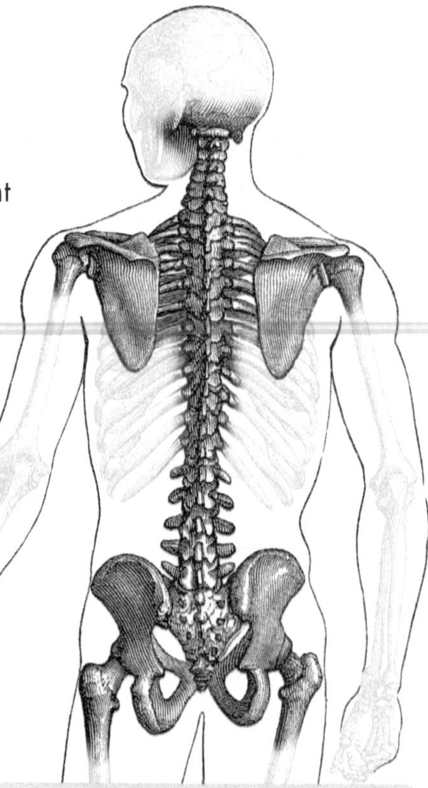

COMFORTABLE SEAT

Intention - To find a position that you can take at any time or place to connect within.

The key components to finding your "Comfortable Seat" are simple: Find a position that you can sit in with your spine straight for at least 5-10 minutes without squirming. Ultimately this position should be one that cultivates a state of peace.

How to get into position: Come into a kneeling position.

Root your sit bones into your heels as you expand and lengthen your spine up.

Release your tailbone down toward the floor

Gently draw in the area 1" below your navel.

Lift your inner sternum up, as you soften your lower ribs downward.

Glide your skull backward so that your ears align with your shoulders.

Settle in.

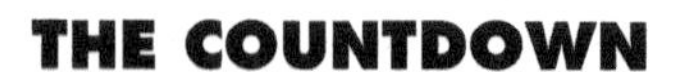

THE COUNTDOWN

Purpose - To train the mind to concentrate its attention on one object without losing focus.

Find a Comfortable Seat. Without altering your breath, tune into your inhale and exhale.

On the exhale, mentally say "fifty".

On the inhale, mentally say "forty-nine".

Count down until you reach "zero"

SPINAL BREATHING

Intention - To bring awareness and breath into every vertebra of the spine.

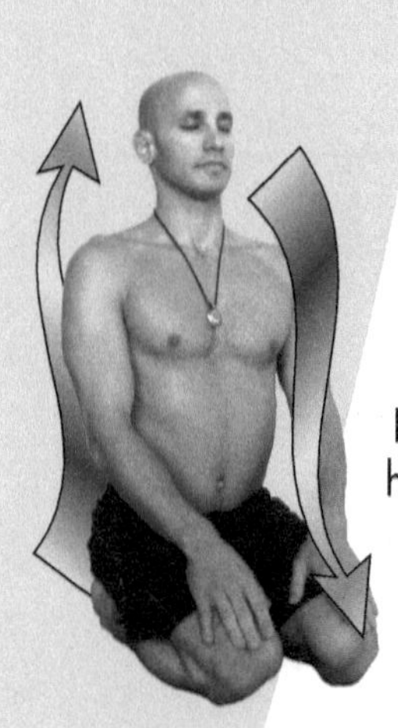

Find a Comfortable Seat. Without altering your breath, tune into your inhale and exhale.

Bring your breath awareness into your tailbone/coccyx.

Bring your breath awareness into your sacrum.

Bring your breath awareness into your lumbar spine/ solar plexus.

Bring your breath awareness into your thoracic spine/ heart center.

Bring your breath awareness into your cervical spine/ throat center.

Bring your breath awareness into the area where your skull meets your spine.

Bring your breath awareness down your spine in reverse order.

ENERGIZING SEQUENCES

"Feel the Flow"

Life begins on an inhale and ends on an exhale. Take a moment... or ten... to tune into the rhythm of your breath. By slowing down... pausing... concentrating... and breathing in your body, you have the power to decrease the stress response and create new positive pathways in your brain.

For centuries, humans have controlled the fluctuation of the breath and have been rewarded with increased health and vitality.

So, find a quiet space... create for yourself a comfortable seat... and tap into the rise and fall of your breath.

SINGLE NOSTRIL BREATHING • Left Side

Intention - To activate the right side of the brain which will induce a calming or relaxing effect.

Find a comfortable seat.

With your right hand, flex the right index and middle finger into your thumb pad.

Cover your right nostril with your thumb.

Exhale slowly through your left nostril. Then breathe naturally and maximally into your left nostril.

Hold for a second, and exhale through left nostril.

Repeat 20 inhales and exhales.

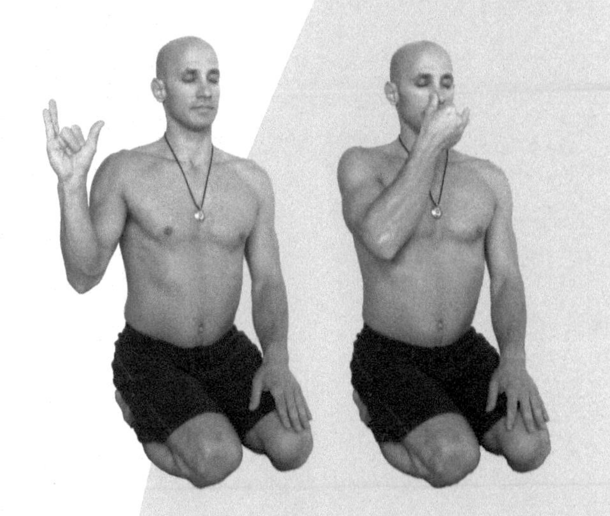

SINGLE NOSTRIL BREATHING • Right Side

Intention - To activate the left side of the brain which will induce a stimulating or energizing effect.

Find a comfortable seat.

With your right hand, flex the right index and middle finger into your thumb pad.

Cover your left nostril with your ring and little finger.

Breathe naturally and maximally into your right nostril.

Hold for a second, and exhale through the right nostril.

Repeat 20 inhales and exhales.

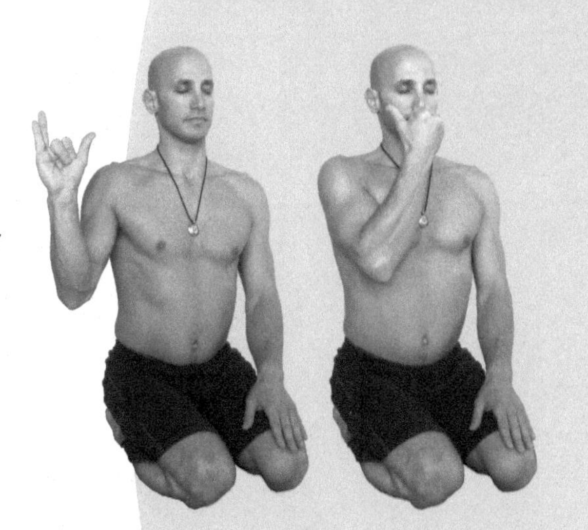

ALTERNATE NOSTRIL BREATHING

Intention - To create optimum function on both sides of the brain.

Find a comfortable seat.

With your right hand, flex the right index and middle finger into your thumb pad.

Cover your right nostril with your ring and little finger.

Exhale slowly through your right nostril. Then breathe naturally and maximally into your left nostril.

Hold for a second, cover your left nostril, open your right nostril, and exhale through the right nostril.

Inhale through the right nostril. Pause. Cover your right nostril, and exhale through the left nostril. This completes a full cycle.

Repeat 20 times.

NOTE: Alternate nostril breathing should not be practiced if you have a cold or if your nasal passages are blocked in an any way.

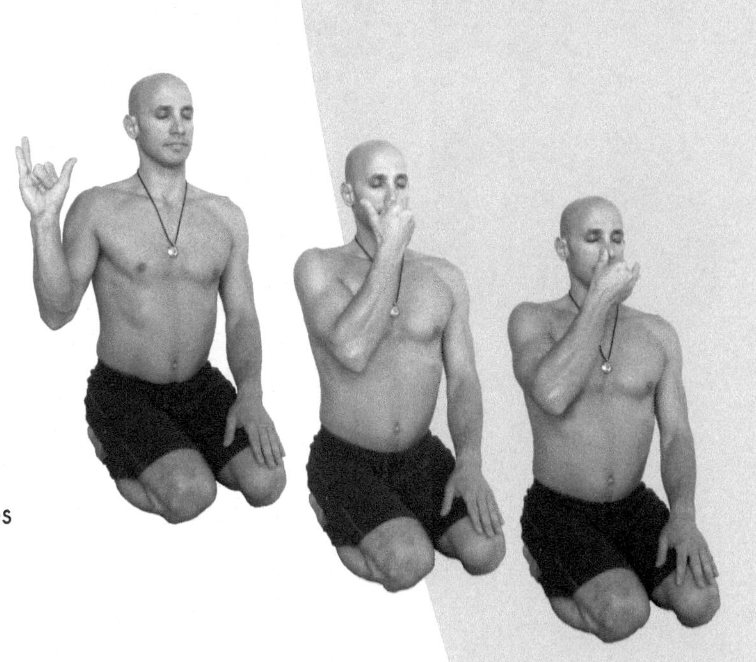

HIGH VIBRATIONAL WORDS • Concentration

Intention - To invigorate your body mind with powerful words to create high vibrational images in your mind's eye. In order to combat fatigue and strengthen your mental thought processing, play this alphabet game. Break yourself out of your negative thought loops. Break it into your mind by thinking positively!

How to:

- You can be in any position, sitting, standing, lying down, or engaging in yoga or exercise.
- Come up with a high vibration word for each letter of the alphabet.
- If you are exercising try doing a squat for each letter/word. If you are feeling inspired, try doing a pull up for each letter/word.
- If you can't think of a word, you may have to hold the squat for a long time!
- Have fun and get creative!

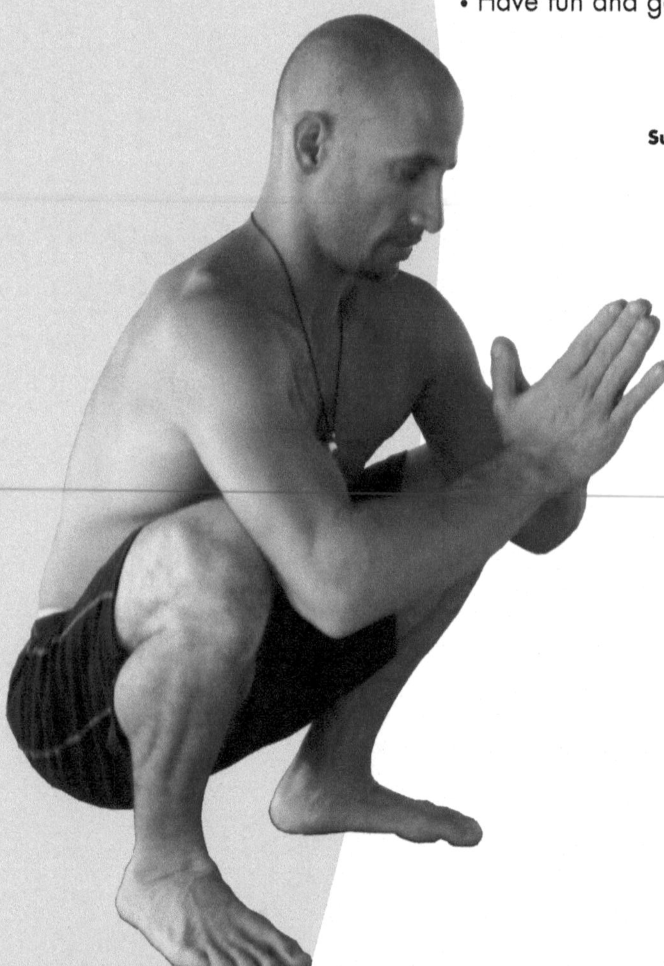

Suggestions:

A Authentic
B Boldness
C Commitment
D Dedication
E Eloquent
F Fertile
G Generous
H Heightened
I Integrity
J Jovial
K Kabbalah
L Love
M Magnetic
N Nectar
O Om
P Passion
Q Quintessential
R Rejuvenate
S Stabilized
T Tenacity
U Understanding
V Victorious
W Willpower
X Xenodochial
Y Yoke
Z Zoom

AFFIRMATIONS • Mental Motivation

"In your daily life, play a game of prosperity. Act, talk, think and feel like you already have what you desire. When you exercise a muscle, it becomes stronger. Plant and nurture a seed, and it grows. What you concentrate on expands. Realize that you choose the future with your thots."

Dr. Fred Schofield

How To:

Read your affirmations **three** times per day and you will bathe your mind with concepts of prosperity.

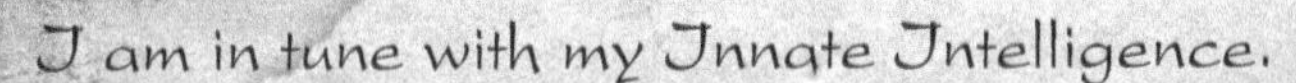

I am in tune with my Innate Intelligence.

My Educated Intelligence communicates easily with my Innate Intelligence.

All the cells of my body are working perfectly.

My body has tremendous healing powers!

My body recreates itself with the greatest of ease.

I tap into my healing reservoir.

I convert disruptive thoughts, behaviors, and actions into constructive thoughts, behaviors, and actions.

I love to take deep breaths.

My body loves to move.

I am able to concentrate my mind's power onto anything I focus on.

I am able to access the wellspring of healing in my body at all times.

I am thankful for the body I have.

I love chiropractic adjustments.

My body receives chiropractic adjustments with the greatest of ease.

I have a flexible and strong spine.

I am responsible for my health.

I am a soldier of health.

I am healthy in mind and body.

People respect me because of the healthy choices I make for myself and my family.

My will power is strong. I can accomplish anything.

I have tremendous endurance and energy.

I reach my goals because of my determination.

I am a warrior.

I am a survivor.

I am successful.

REFERENCE & CREDITS

GLOSSARY

asana • *A posture or yogic pose. Classically defined as a seat.*

jalandara bandha • *A yogic procedure of locking the chin to the breastbone.*

mula bandha • *A yogic procedure involving contracting the muscles of the perineum resulting in a "rectal lock".*

sun salutation • *A series of twelve yoga postures performed in a single graceful flow with each movement coordinated with the breath; also called "surya namaskar".*

uddiyana bandha • *A yogic procedure involving pulling in the abdominal muscles and organs resulting in an abdominal lock.*

vertebral subluxation • *WORLD HEALTH ORGANIZATION DEFINITION:*
A lesion or dysfunction in a joint or motion segment in which alignment, movement integrity and/or physiological function are altered, although contact between joint surfaces remains intact. It is essentially a functional entity, which may influence biomechanical and neural integrity.

vinyasa • *A specifc set of movements linked with breath in a prescribed manner.*

BOOKS FOR WISDOM, VITALITY, INSIGHT AND INSPIRATION

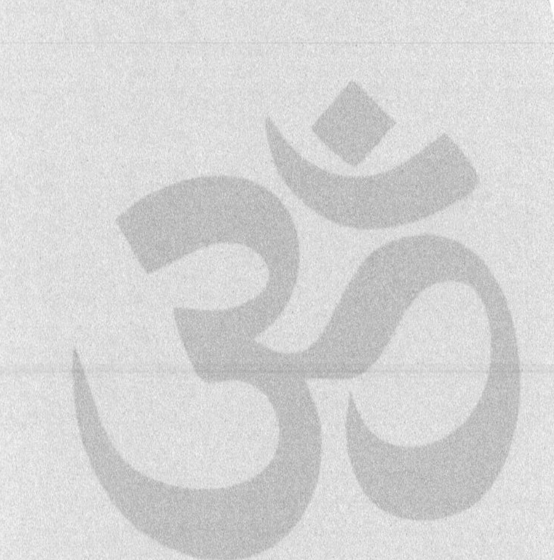

Batmanghelidj, M.D, F.. ***Your Body's Many Cries for Water.*** London: Global Health Solutions, Inc., 2008.

Books, Brooline, and Daniel R. Kamen. ***The Well Adjusted Dog: Canine Chiropractic Methods You Can Do.*** Cambridge, Massachussetts: Brookline Books, 1997.

Carillo, Anthony, and Eric Neuhaus. ***Iron Yoga: Combine Yoga and Strength Training for Weight Loss and Total Body Fitness.*** Emmaus, Pa.: Rodale Books, 2005.

Carlisi, Anthony Prem. ***Only Way Out Is In: A Modern Day Yogi's Commentary on the Synergy of Ashtanga Yoga, Ayurveda, and Tantra.*** unknown: Dream Weavers International, 2007.

Cousens, Gabriel. ***Spiritual Nutrition: Six Foundations for Spiritual Life and the Awakening of Kundalini.*** California: North Atlantic Books, 2005.

Deitch, Jason, and Bob Hoffman. ***Discover Wellness: How Staying Healthy Can Make You Rich.*** unknown: Center Path Publishing, 2007.

Gurmukh, and Cathryn Michon. ***The Eight Human Talents.*** New York: Collins Living, 2000.

Hamilton, Laird. ***Force of Nature: Mind, Body, Soul (And, of Course, Surfing).*** Emmaus, Pa.: Rodale Books, 2008.

Jaffe, Dennis T.. ***Healing from Within.*** New York: Fireside, 1986.

Kessel, Brent. ***It's Not About the Money: Unlock Your Money Type to Achieve Spiritual and Financial Abundance.*** New York: Harperone, 2008.

Lee, Bruce, and M. Uyehara. ***Bruce Lee's Fighting Method: The Complete Edition.*** San Francisco: Black Belt Communications, 2008.

Leonard, George. ***Mastery: The Keys to Success and Long-Term Fulfillment (Plume).*** New York: Plume, 1992.

Lipton, Bruce H.. ***The Biology of Belief: Unleashing the Power of Consciousness, Matter, & Miracles.*** Carlsbad: Hay House, 2008.

Marcus, Bach. ***The Chiropractic Story.*** unknown: De Vorss & Co., 1968.

Marinoff, Lou. ***The Therapy for the Sane.*** New York: Bloomsbury USA, 2004.

Perlmutter, Jenness Cortez, and Leonard Perlmutter. ***The Heart And Science of Yoga: A Blueprint for Peace, Happiness And Freedom from Fear.*** New York: Ami Publishers, 2005.

Plasker, Dr. Eric. ***The 100 Year Lifestyle: Dr Plasker's Breakthrough Solution for Living Your Best Life - Every Day of Your Life!.*** Avon, MA: Listen & Live Audio, Inc., 2007.

Pollan, Michael. ***In Defense of Food: The Myth of Nutrition and the Pleasures of Eating.*** New York: Penguin Press HC, The, 2007.

Powers, Ryan, and Michael Wissot. ***The 10 People Who Suck - A Positive Prescription for Improving Communication in the Workplace.*** Tacoma: City Hall Publishing, 2007.

Ramaswami, Srivatsa. ***The Complete Book of Vinyasa Yoga: The Authoritative Presentation-Based on 30 Years of Direct Study Under the Legendary Yoga Teacher Krishnamacha.*** New York and Washington D.C.: Da Capo Press, 2005.

Remnick, David. ***King of the World: Muhammed Ali and the Rise of an American Hero.*** New York: Vintage, 1999.

Schefter, Adam, and Mike Shanahan. ***Think Like A Champion: Building Success One Victory at a Time.*** London: Collins, 2000.

Schiffmann, Erich. ***Yoga: The Spirit and Practice of Moving into Stillness.*** New York: Pocket, 1996.

Sharma, Robin S.. ***Megaliving! : 30 Days to a Perfect Life: The Ultimate Action Plan for Total Mastery of Your Mind, Body & Character.*** Canada: Haunsla Corporation, 1995.

Spielman, Ed. ***Spiritual Journey of Joseph L.*** Greenstein: The Mighty Atom. Hillsboro, Oregon: First Glance Books, 1988.

Talbot, Michael. ***The Holographic Universe.*** New York: Harper Perennial, 1992.

Taylor, Jill Bolte. ***My Stroke of Insight: A Brain Scientist's Personal Journey.*** New York: Viking Adult, 2008.

Vivekananda, Swami. ***RAJA YOGA: Vendanta Philosophy; Being Lectures By the Swami Vivekananda with Patanjali's Aphorisms, Commentaries and a Glossary of Terms.*** Chicago: Brentano's, 1927.

Yogananda, Paramahansa. ***Autobiography of a Yogi.*** Los Angeles: Self-Realization Fellowship Publishers, 2006.

Yogananda, Paramahansa. ***Scientific Healing Affirmations: Theory and Practice of Concentration.*** Calcutta: Self-Realization Fellowship, 1958.

ACKNOWLEDGMENTS & GRATITUDE

This manifesto is stuffed with original ideas - some of them my own, some of them channeled, most from my teachers. I am deeply grateful and indebted to all those whose teachings I have raided, memorized and incorporated into this manifesto.

There are so many people to thank for inspiring me to create this manifesto. I'll start with my creators and parents...thanks Mom (Margie) and Dad (Joe)! To my grandparents who gave me all the love and support a grandkid could ask for. Special thanks to my sister, Allison, my lifelong best friend and confidant, and her husband Todd. Thank you to Jo, my beautiful girlfriend and teacher. Thank you to my Aunts Carolyn, Dorothy, and Marsha, and my Uncles Ethan, Dr. Scotty, and Barry. To my cousins, Robyn, Jason, Dr. Mike (in 2009), Adam, Dan, Karen, and Gil and the rest of the mishpacha.

Special shout out to my teachers: First my chiropractic mentors: Dr. Paul Webber (my first chiropractor!), Dr. Arno Burnier, Dr. Fred Schofield, Dr. Ron Oberstein, Dr. Mindy Pelz, Dr. Shelley Roth, Dr. Richard Warner, Dr. Robert Cooperstein, Dr. Richard De Sarbo, Dr. Bill De Moss, Dr. Brian Porteous, Dr. Jon Baker, Dr. Hans Freericks, and last, but not least, Drs. B.J. and D.D. Palmer.

Special gratitude to my yoga teachers...Marti Foster, Erich Schiffmann, Saul David Raye, Chuck Miller, Jo Tastula (again), Matthew Cohen, Hala Khouri, and Raghavan.

Deep gratitude to my chiropractic school friends who gave up their body and mind to learn how to adjust one another: Dr. Travis Meier, Dr. Phillip Grivas, Dr. Brian Austin, Dr. Chris Chalrton, & Dr. Amber Kirk.

Thank you to my friends who selflessly went face down on my portable chiropractic table to receive their first ever adjustment from me while in chiropractic school. The thousands of people I have adjusted thank you too! Bryan Pozzo, Tucker Spear, Mark Hochberg, Tom Hudack, Dan Bochner and Todd Bochner to name a few.

Thank you to my assistants Joann, Darla, Nickey, and Tracey. You are the muscles and organs of The Life Center Chiropractic. Thank you to my old assistants Jasmine, Marcia, and Lisa. Your hard work and dedication is not forgotten.

Special thanks to the woman behind the manifesto, Yoli Hodde, whose design and photography brought it to life!

Thank you to my extra eyes who helped proof this book: Felicia Marie Tomasko, Brian Maser, Kaia Van Zandt, Cindy Knight, Dani Katz, and Norm Larson.

There are so many other people to thank...in the event that you were left off this list, please email me your name and you will be added in the next printing!

"Yo, Adrian, we did it...
We did it."

Rocky Balboa

NOTES

wobble chair

zero gravity chair to sit/write in

NOTES

Dr. James Chestnut

NOTES